Renal Cookbook And Diet Guide

2 BOOKS IN 1 - The Exhaustive, Complete and Effective Meal Plan For Newly Diagnosed Made By Much Low Sodium, Potassium, and Phosphorus Recipes To Make You Eat And Feel Healthier | +200 Recipes

Elizabeth Cook

© Copyright 2020 - All rights reserved.

The content contained within this book may not be reproduced, duplicated or transmitted without direct written permission from the author or the publisher. Under no circumstances will any blame or legal responsibility be held against the publisher, or author, for any damages, reparation, or monetary loss due to the information contained within this book. Either directly or indirectly.

Legal Notice:

This book is copyright protected. This book is only for personal use. You cannot amend, distribute, sell, use, quote or paraphrase any part, or the content within this book, without the consent of the author or publisher.

Disclaimer Notice:

Please note the information contained within this document is for educational and entertainment purposes only. All effort has been executed to present accurate, up to date, and reliable, complete information. No warranties of any kind are declared or implied. Readers acknowledge that the author is not engaging in the rendering of legal, financial, medical or professional advice. The content within this book has been derived from various sources. Please consult a licensed professional before attempting any techniques outlined in this book.

By reading this document, the reader agrees that under no circumstances is the author responsible for any losses, direct or indirect, which are incurred as a result of the use of information contained within this document, including, but not limited to, errors, omissions, or inaccuracies.

TABLE OF CONTENTS

RENAL DIET

INTRODUCTION	12
CHAPTER ONE: UNDERSTANDING HOW THE KIDNEY FUNCTIONS	13
Kidney Anatomy	13
Kidney Functions	13
Additional Information	14
CHAPTER TWO: UNDERSTANDING KIDNEY DISEASE	15
Stages of Chronic Kidney Failure	16
Kidney Diseases—Causes, Symptoms, Diagnosis, and Treatment	18
CHAPTER THREE: BENEFITS OF FOLLOWING A RENAL DIET	20
Why Is It So Important to Follow a Meal Plan?	20
Fundamentals of the Renal Diet	20
What Is the Difference Between Kidney Diets?	24
Special Dietary Concerns	25
CHAPTER FOUR: HOW TO IMPROVE KIDNEY FUNCTION	26
Eat Healthily	26
Drink Healthily	27
Weight Control and Regular Exercise	27
The Emergence of Kidney Disease	28
How to Avoid Dialysis	28
Steps to Control Chronic Kidney Failure	29
CHAPTER FIVE: FOODS TO AVOID IF YOU HAVE BAD KIDNEY	31
Cola Soda	32
Avocados	32
Canned Food	32
Wholemeal Bread	33
Integral Rice	33
Bananas	33
Dairy Products	33
Oranges and Orange Juice	34
Processed Meats	34
Pickles, Olives, and Sauce	34
Apricots	35
Potatoes and Sweet Potatoes	35
Tomatoes	35
Packaged, Instant, and Prepared Meals	36
Swiss Chard, Spinach, and Beet Greens	36

DATES, RAISINS, AND PLUMS	36
PRETZELS, CHIPS, AND COOKIES	36
BEST FOODS FOR PEOPLE WITH KIDNEY DISEASE	37
DAILY TIPS TO BOOST YOUR KIDNEY FUNCTION	41

CHAPTER SIX: DIET FOR CHRONIC KIDNEY DISEASE — 42

HIGH-CALORIE INTAKE	42
HIGH-CALORIE INTAKE	42
CARBOHYDRATE	42
LIPIDS	43
PROTEIN RESTRICTION	43
WATER INTAKE	43
HELPFUL TIPS TO REDUCE WATER INTAKE	44
SALT RESTRICTION (SODIUM)	45
PRACTICAL ADVICE TO REDUCE YOUR SALT INTAKE	46
POTASSIUM RESTRICTION	47
THE RESTRICTIVE PHOSPHORUS DIET	49
DESIGNING A DAILY DIET	50

CHAPTER SEVEN: 7-DAY PLAN: WHAT TO EAT TO DETOXIFY YOUR KIDNEYS FAST — 51

KIDNEYS DETOX DAY 1	52
KIDNEYS CLEAN DAY 2	52
KIDNEYS CLEAN DAY 3	52
KIDNEYS CLEAN DAY 4	53
KIDNEYS CLEAN DAY 5	53
KIDNEYS CLEAN DAY 6	53
KIDNEYS CLEAN DAY 7	54
MYTHS AND FACTS ABOUT KIDNEY DISEASE	54

RENAL DIET COOKBOOK FOR BEGINNERS

INTRODUCTION — 58

CHAPTER 1: UNDERSTANDING KIDNEY DISEASE — 59

WHAT DO THE KIDNEYS DO?	59
WHAT CAUSES KIDNEY DISEASE?	59
TREATMENT PLANS FOR CHRONIC KIDNEY DISEASE (CKD)	60

CHAPTER 2: THE CAUSES OF RENAL FAILURE — 62

SYMPTOMS OF KIDNEY DISEASE?	63
DIAGNOSE WITH KIDNEY DISEASE	63

CHAPTER 3: WHAT YOU CAN EAT, WHAT TO AVOID — 65

FOODS YOU NEED	65
FOODS YOU NEED TO AVOID	66
RENAL DIET SHOPPING LIST	67

CHAPTER 4: MEAL PLAN	**71**
CHAPTER 5: BREAKFAST	**73**
Easy Turnip Puree	73
Green lettuce Bacon Breakfast Bake	74
Healthy Green lettuce Tomato Muffins	75
Chicken Egg Breakfast Muffins	76
Breakfast Egg Salad	77
Vegetable Tofu Scramble	78
Cheese Coconut Pancakes	79
Cheesy Scrambled Eggs with Fresh Herbs	80
Coconut Breakfast Smoothie	81
Turkey and Green lettuce Scramble on Melba Toast	82
Vegetable Omelet	83
Mexican Style Burritos	84
Bulgur, Couscous and Buckwheat Cereal	85
Sweet Pancakes	86
Breakfast Smoothie	87
Buckwheat and Grapefruit Porridge	88
Egg and Veggie Muffins	89
Salad with Vinaigrette	90
Salad with Lemon Dressing	91
Shrimp with Salsa	92
Pesto Pork Chops	93
Turkey Burgers	94
CHAPTER 6: LUNCH	**96**
Dolmas Wrap	96
Salad al Tonno	97
Arlecchino Rice Salad	97
Sauteed Chickpea and Lentil Mix	98
Crazy Japanese Potato and Beef Croquettes	99
Traditional Black Bean Chili	100
Green Palak Paneer	101
Cucumber Sandwich	102
Pizza Pitas	103
Lettuce Wraps with Chicken	104
Turkey Pinwheels	105
Chicken Tacos	106
Tuna Twist	107
Ciabatta Rolls with Chicken Pesto	108
Marinated Shrimp Pasta Salad	108
Peanut Butter and Jelly Grilled Sandwich	109
Grilled Onion and Pepper Jack Grilled Cheese Sandwich	110
Crispy Lemon Chicken	111
Mexican Steak Tacos	112

Beer Pork Ribs	113
Mexican Chorizo Sausage	114
Eggplant Casserole	115
Pizza with Chicken and Pesto	116
Shrimp Quesadilla	117
Grilled Corn on the Cob	118
Couscous with Veggies	119
Easy Egg Salad	120
Cauliflower Rice and Coconut	120
Kale and Garlic Platter	121
Blistered Beans and Almond	122
Cucumber Soup	123
Eggplant Salad	123
Cajun Crab	124
Mushroom Pork Chops	125
Caramelized Pork Chops	126
Mediterranean Pork	127
Ground Beef and Bell Peppers	128
Spiced Up Pork Chops	129
Juicy Salmon Dish	130
Platter-O-Brussels	131
Almond Chicken	132
BlackBerry Chicken Wings	133
Aromatic Carrot Cream	133
Mushrooms Velvet Soup	134
Easy Lettuce Wraps	136
Spaghetti with Pesto	137
Vegetable Casserole	138
Appetizing Rice Salad	139
Spiced Wraps	140
Rump Roast	141

CHAPTER 7: DINNER — 142

Beef Kabobs with Pepper	142
One-Pot Beef Roast	143
Cabbage and Beef Fry	144
California Pork Chops	145
Caribbean Turkey Curry	146
Chicken Fajitas	146
Chicken Veronique	147
Chicken and Apple Curry	148
London Broil	149
Sirloin with Squash and Pineapple	150
Slow-Cooked BBQ Beef	151
Lemon Sprouts	152
Lemon and Broccoli Platter	153

Chicken Liver Stew	153
Simple Lamb Chops	154
Chicken and Mushroom Stew	155
Roasted Carrot Soup	156
Garlic and Butter-Flavored Cod	157
Tilapia Broccoli Platter	157
Parsley Scallops	158
Blackened Chicken	159
Spicy Paprika Lamb Chops	160
Mushroom and Olive Sirloin Steak	160
Parsley and Chicken Breast	161
Simple Mustard Chicken	162
Golden Eggplant Fries	163
Very Wild Mushroom Pilaf	164
Sporty Baby Carrots	164
Saucy Garlic Greens	165
Garden Salad	166
Spicy Cabbage Dish	167
Extreme Balsamic Chicken	168
Enjoyable Green lettuce and Bean Medley	169
Tantalizing Cauliflower and Dill Mash	170
Peas Soup	171
Minty Lamb Stew	172
Spicy Mushroom Stir-Fry	172
Curried Veggies and Rice	174
Spicy Veggie Pancakes	175
Egg and Veggie Fajitas	176
Vegetable Biryani	176
Creamy Tuna Salad	178
Creamy Mushroom Soup	179
Pork Soup	180
Thai Chicken Soup	181
Tasty Pumpkin Soup	181
Easy Zucchini Soup	182
Quick Tomato Soup	183
Spicy Chicken Soup	184
Shredded Pork Soup	185
Creamy Chicken Green lettuce Soup	185
Shrimp Paella	186
Salmon & Pesto Salad	187
Baked Fennel & Garlic Sea Bass	189
Lemon, Garlic, Cilantro Tuna and Rice	190
Cod & Green Bean Risotto	191
Sardine Fish Cakes	192
4-Ingredients Salmon Fillet	193
Spanish Cod in Sauce	194

    Salmon Baked in Foil with Fresh Thyme   195
    Poached Halibut in Orange Sauce   196

CHAPTER 8: SNACK RECIPES   198

    Veggie Snack   198
    Healthy Spiced Nuts   199
    Roasted Asparagus   200
    Low-Fat Mango Salsa   201
    Vinegar & Salt Kale   202
    Carrot and Parsnips French Fries   203
    Apple & Strawberry Snack   203
    Candied Macadamia Nuts   204
    Cinnamon Apple Fries   205
    Lemon Pops   206
    Easy No-Bake Coconut Cookies   206
    Roasted Chili-Vinegar Peanuts   207
    Popcorn with Sugar and Spice   208
    Eggplant and Chickpea Bites   209
    Baba Ghanouj   210
    Baked Pita Fries   211
    Herbal Cream Cheese Tartines   212
    Mixes of Snacks   212
    Spicy Crab Dip   213
    Baked Apples with Cherries and Walnuts   214
    Easy Peach Crumble   215

CHAPTER 9: 40 RECIPES FOR THOSE WHO HAVE DIALYSIS: BREAKFAST   216

    Breakfast Salad from Grains and Fruits   216
    French toast with Applesauce   217
    Bagels Made Healthy   218
    Cornbread with Southern Twist   219
    Grandma's Pancake Special   220
    Pasta with Indian Lentils   221
    Shrimp Bruschetta   221
    Strawberry Muesli   222
    Yogurt Bulgur   223
    Mozzarella Cheese Omelet   224

CHAPTER 10: LUNCH   226

    Couscous and Sherry Vinaigrette   226
    Persian Chicken   227
    Ratatouille   228
    Jicama Noodles   229
    Crack Slaw   230
    Vegan Chili   231
    Chow Mein   232

MUSHROOM TACOS	233
LIME GREEN LETTUCE AND CHICKPEAS SALAD	234
FRIED RICE WITH KALE	235
STIR-FRIED GINGERY VEGGIES	235

CHAPTER 11: DINNER 237

FISH EN' PAPILLOTE	237
PESTO PASTA SALAD	238
BARLEY BLUEBERRY SALAD	239
PASTA WITH CREAMY BROCCOLI SAUCE	240
ASPARAGUS FRIED RICE	241
BEEF AND CHILI STEW	242
STICKY PULLED BEEF OPEN SANDWICHES	243
HERBY BEEF STROGANOFF AND FLUFFY RICE	245
CHUNKY BEEF AND POTATO SLOW ROAST	246
SPICED LAMB BURGERS	247
PORK LOINS WITH LEEKS	248
THE KALE AND GREEN LETTUCE SOUP	249
JAPANESE ONION SOUP	250
AMAZING BROCCOLI AND CAULIFLOWER SOUP	251

CHAPTER 12: SNACKS 253

LEMON THINS	253
SNICKERDOODLE CHICKPEA BLONDIES	254
CHOCOLATE CHIA SEED PUDDING	255
CHOCOLATE-MINT TRUFFLES	256
PERSONAL MANGO PIES	257
GRILLED PEACH SUNDAES	258
BLUEBERRY SWIRL CAKE	259
PEANUT BUTTER COOKIES	260
DELICIOUSLY GOOD SCONES	261
MIXED BERRY COBBLER	261
BLUEBERRY ESPRESSO BROWNIES	262
COFFEE BROWNIES	263
CONCLUSION	**265**

RENAL DIET

The Definitive Guide to Manage This Disease. How to Improve the Renal Function and How to Avoid Dialysis. What to Eat and Not, Daily Quantities to Get Potassium, Phosphorus, Fluid, and Sodium

Elizabeth Cook

INTRODUCTION

The kidney is a wonderful organ that is important to your body's health through waste the elimination and excretion. Although the primary function of a kidney is the purifying function, the kidneys play a major role in regulating the blood pressure, fluid volume, and electrical concentrations in the body.

However, nearly everyone has two kidneys at birth, but in the last few years, the human body can function with only one kidney, increasing in patients with diabetes and highly bloated pain. It enables us to help people to become aware of this plague and to explain diseases better.

This book will be about kidneys, disease prevention, and the value of early treatment. The aim is to help patients better understand and manage the disease of the kidneys when it occurs.

If you experience chronic diseases such as high blood pressure, diabetes, heart and kidney disease, what you eat is crucial. Patients suffering from chronic kidney disease normally have a diet tailored by their doctor. This diet will continue to change constantly, depending on the state of the renal disease. Be sure that you keep a journal of what you eat every day as a patient with renal disease. This is essential for your nutritionist. It is also important to invest in a scale every morning to monitor your weight. In most cases, individuals with chronic kidney disease have to gain weight or retain weight.

If you lose too much bodyweight, your dietician may add extra calories to your diet. When you eat more calories than your body spends, you get a weight gain. That is why most people are obese and overweight. On the other hand, your dietician can guide you safely to reduce your daily calorie intake and increase your activity if you gain too much weight. Additional operations consume the energy of the mire.

It is a matter of concern that you can quickly gain weight, as it may be a sign that your body has too much fluid. Doctors specifically seek weight gain along with swelling, shortness of breath, and increased blood pressure. For your overall condition and feeling, when you have chronic kidney disease, it is important to get the right amount of protein. When building muscles, repairing tissues and fighting infections, your body needs the right amount of protein. If your protein levels are not adequate, you may be advised by your doctor to use a diet that has a controlled amount of protein.

This reduces the amount of waste in your blood and may make your kidneys work longer. Protein can be taken individually from two sources, namely plant and animal sources. Animal sources include eggs, fish, chicken, red meat, milk and cheese. Plants are also included in vegetables and grains.

Besides protein, you need to have other significant nutrients in your diet. Nutrients are available that you need in the right amount to be in your best daily condition. Sodium is one of these. A combination of kidney, high blood pressure, and sodium is often found. It is important to limit sodium in your diet to keep your blood pressure under control. Control of your high blood pressure is of primary importance when you suffer from kidney disease. This means eating fewer salt foods or salt alternatives.

CHAPTER ONE:
UNDERSTANDING HOW
THE KIDNEY FUNCTIONS

The balance of the internal chemistry of our bodies is largely due to the kidneys' work. Our survival depends on these vital organs functioning normally.

The kidneys are responsible for four functions in the body:

- Elimination of toxins from the blood by a filtration system;
- Regulation of blood and bone formation;
- Blood pressure regulation;
- Control of the delicate chemical and liquid balance of the body.

The kidneys are vital organs, as essential to our life as our heart or our lungs. However, they remain poorly understood, just like the diseases that affect them. These so-called silent diseases are, in a good number of cases, diagnosed too late, while early and appropriate management can slow or even stop their development. When faced with kidney failure and its treatments, getting informed and understanding is essential.

Kidney Anatomy
Each person normally has two kidneys, but one kidney is enough to live. The kidneys are flattened, ovoid, and complex functioning organs. Contrary to popular belief that the kidneys are located in the lower back, they are located just below the rib cage (at the last ribs' height).

Kidney Functions
The Main Purpose of the Kidneys
The main function of the kidneys is to remove water and water-soluble substances (end products of metabolism) from the body. The excretory function is closely related to the regulation function of the ionic and acid-base balance of the internal environment of the body. Hormones control both functions. Also, the kidneys perform an endocrine function, taking a direct part in synthesizing many hormones. Finally, the kidneys are involved in intermediate metabolic processes, especially in gluconeogenesis and cleavage of peptides and amino acids.

A very large volume of blood passes through the kidneys: 1500 litres per day. From this volume, 180l of primary urine is filtered. Then the volume of primary urine is significantly reduced due to the reabsorption of water; thus, the daily output of urine is 0.5–2.0 litres.

Process of Urination

The kidney's functional (and structural) unit is the nephron; there are approximately 1 million nephrons in the human kidney. The nephrotic urination process consists of three phases:

- **Ultrafiltration (glomerular or glomerular filtration).** In the glomeruli of the renal corpuscles, primary urine is formed from blood plasma during ultrafiltration, isosmotic with blood plasma. The pores through which the plasma is filtered have an effective average diameter of 2.9nm. With this pore size, all blood plasma components with a molecular weight up to 5 kDa freely pass through the membrane. Substances with M <65 kDa partially pass through the pores, and only large molecules (M> 65 kDa) are retained by the pores and do not enter the primary urine. Since most blood plasma proteins have a fairly high molecular weight (M> 54 kDa) and are negatively charged; they are retained by the glomerular basement membrane. The protein content in the ultrafiltration is insignificant.

- **Reabsorption.** Primary urine is concentrated (about 100 times the original volume) due to the reverse filtration of water. At the same time, by the mechanism of active transport, practically all low-molecular substances, especially glucose, amino acids, as well as most electrolytes (inorganic and organic ions) are reabsorbed in the tubules. The reabsorption of amino acids is carried out using group-specific transport systems (carriers), with a defect associated with several genetically determined hereditary diseases (cystinosis, glycosuria, Hartnup's syndrome).

Additional Information

- **Metabolism.** Concentration and selective transport processes are energy-intensive. The required ATP is synthesized through the oxidation of fatty acids, ketone bodies, and some amino acids, and to a lesser, extent lactate, glycerol, citrate, and glucose, which are found in the blood. In the kidneys, just like in the liver, the process of gluconeogenesis can take place. The substrates are the carbon skeletons of glucogenic amino acids, the nitrogen of which ammonia is used to regulate urine pH. In the kidneys, enzymes of the cleavage of peptides and amino acids' metabolism are found with high activity (for example, amino acid oxidase, amine oxidase, and glutaminase).

- **Renal clearance (renal cleansing).** This is the most used indicator by which the rate of renal excretion of certain substances from the blood is determined. It is defined as the volume of blood plasma purified from a specific substance per unit of time. The clearance of inulin, polyfructazan with $M \approx 6kDa$, which is well filtered, but does not undergo active reabsorption and secretion, serves as an indicator of the glomerular filtration rate. The normal value of the glomerular filtration rate, determined by inulin, is 120ml/min.

CHAPTER TWO:
UNDERSTANDING KIDNEY DISEASE

Only in the United States, kidney conditions are estimated to affect 31 million people, and at a worldwide level, one of each ten people has a kidney disease. Kidney disease, also known as renal disease, is the overall term for damage, reducing kidney function. Chronic kidney disease (CKD) occurs when the kidneys can no longer clear and function with toxins and wastes from the blood. This can happen suddenly or overtime. There are five different phases of chronic kidney disease (CKD).

Our two kidneys every day philtre approximately 120 to 150 quarters of kidney blood and produce approximately 1 to 2 quarts of waste urine and extra fluid.2 Healthy kidneys help regulate blood pressure, remove rubbish and water, signal that your body is making red blood cells and help control childhood growth.

The chronic renal failure or uremia is the kidneys' inability to produce urine or fabricate low quality ("like water") since it has not been removed enough toxic waste. Although some patients continue to urinate, most cannot. However, the important thing is not the quantity, but the composition or quality of the urine.

The kidneys are two "bean-shaped" organs located in the dorsal wall of the body on the sides of the spine. They are brown, weigh about 150-grams each, and are about 12 centimetres long, 6 centimetres wide, and 3 centimetres thick. In the upper part, each kidney has an endocrine gland attached (it produces vital substances inside the body) called the adrenal gland.

The kidneys are the "purifiers" where the blood is filtered and cleaned. They produce urine, which contains water, toxins, and salts that the blood has been collecting throughout the body, and that has to be eliminated. They also intervene in other activities such as reproduction because they make sex hormones; regulate the amount of phosphorus and calcium in the bones; they control the tension in the blood vessels, and manufacture substances involved in blood clotting.

Renal insufficiency appears when only 5 per cent of the total kidney or nephron filters work. The basic unit of the kidney is the nephron, of which there are about 1 million in each organ. Each nephron is formed by a component that acts as a filter, the glomerulus, and a transport system, the tubule.

Some of the blood that reaches the kidneys is filtered by the glomerulus and passes through the tubules. Various excretion and reabsorption processes occur, resulting in urine that is eventually removed.

The renal blood flow (RBF or amount of blood reaching the kidney per minute) is approximately 1.1 litres per minute in adults. Of the 0.6 litres of plasma that enter the glomerulus through the arterioles, 20 per cent are filtered, an operation called renal glomerular filtration.

The renal glomerular filtrate is, therefore, the volume of plasma filtered by the kidneys per unit of time. The amount of filtered plasma per day is 135 to 160 litres. To prevent fluid loss, between 98 per cent and 99 per cent of the renal glomerular filtration rate is reabsorbed by the tubules, resulting in the amount of urine removed resulting from between one and two litres per day.

When a kidney disorder occurs, it means that one or more of the renal functions are altered. But not all functions are altered in the same proportion; if, for example, two-thirds of the nephrons cease to function, significant changes may not occur because the remaining nephrons adapt. Likewise, changes in hormonal production may go unnoticed, and then the calculation of renal glomerular filtration is the only way to detect the decrease in the number of nephrons that continue to function.

Stages of Chronic Kidney Failure
An average of 180 litres of blood per day is filtered by the two kidneys, about 90 to 125ml per minute. The rate of glomerular filtration or creatinine clearance is called this. The phases of chronic renal failure are divided by the rate of glomerular filtration, which can be estimated using creatinine levels in the blood. To estimate the degree of functioning of the kidneys from the values of creatinine, several mathematical formulas exist. Nowadays, when creatinine dosage is requested, most laboratories already automatically do this calculation.

Renal failure, with a deterioration of function over the years, is often a progressive illness. The risk of rapid kidney function loss is increased by certain factors, such as poorly controlled diabetes and hypertension.

We have divided the IRC stages as follows:

CKD Stage 1
Patients with creatinine clearance greater than 90 ml/min but any of the above-described diseases (diabetes mellitus, high blood pressure, polycystic kidneys, etc.)

Patients with one or more of these conditions always have some degree of kidney damage that, however, may not yet be reflected in the blood's filtering capacity. They are patients with normal renal function, with no symptoms, but a high risk of deterioration of long-term renal function.

With normal creatinine, but with changes in the urine test, patients also reach this stage, with signs of bleeding or protein loss in the urine.

Stage 2
Patients with creatinine clearance between 60 and 89 ml/min.
This can be called the pre-renal failure stage. They are people with small losses of kidney function, being the earliest stage of kidney failure.

As the kidneys lose function naturally with age, many older people may have slightly reduced kidney function. This drop-in function is simply a sign of the ageing of the kidneys. Therefore, finding older people with criteria for stage II CRF is extremely common. If the patient does not have any disease that attacks the kidneys, such as diabetes or hypertension, this slight kidney function loss does not cause major problems in the medium/long term.

In stage II, the kidney is still able to maintain its basic functions, and blood creatinine is still very close to the normal range. However, it is important to note that these patients are at greater risk of worsening renal function if exposed, for example, to drugs that are toxic to the kidneys, such as anti-inflammatory drugs or contrasts for radiological examinations.

Stage 3
Patients with creatinine clearance between 30 and 59 ml/min.
This is the stage of chronic renal failure that has been declared. Creatinine is already higher than the reference values, and the first disease complications are beginning to develop. The kidney has already decreased its ability to produce erythropoietin, a hormone that controls bone marrow production of red blood cells, causing the patient to develop progressive anaemia.

Bone injury is another issue that is starting to arise. Inadequate renal patients have a disease called renal osteodystrophy, caused by an increase in PTH and a decrease in vitamin D production, a hormone that controls the amount of calcium in the bones and blood. The result is the demineralization of the bones, which are beginning to get weak and sick.

Stage III is the stage in which patients must start treatment and be accompanied by a nephrologist, since from this point on there is usually a relatively rapid progression of renal failure if there is no adequate treatment.

Stage 4
Patients with creatinine clearance between 15 and 29 ml/min.
This is the stage for pre-dialysis. This is when the first symptoms start to appear, and several changes are shown in laboratory tests.

The patient has high phosphorus and PTH levels, established anaemia, low blood pH (increased blood acidity), high potassium levels, weight loss and signs of malnutrition, worsening hypertension, weakened bone levels, increased risk of heart disease, decreased libido, decreased appetite, fatigue, etc.

The patient may not notice weight loss due to fluid retention, as the weight may remain the same or even increase. The patient loses fat and muscle mass but retains fluids, and small edema in the legs may develop.

The patient should already be ready for hemodialysis at this stage, indicating the construction of an arteriovenous fistula.

Stage 5
Patients with a creatinine clearance of less than 15 ml/min.
This is referred to as an end-stage renal failure. The kidney no longer performs basic functions below 15–10 ml/min, and the commencement of dialysis is indicated. At this point that patients, called uremia symptoms, begin to experience symptoms of kidney failure.

If dialysis is not started, the condition progresses. Those who do not die from cardiac arrhythmias may progress with pulmonary edema or mental changes, such as disorientation, seizure crisis, and even coma. Although they are still able to urinate, the volume is not so large, and the patient begins to develop large edema.

Blood pressure is out of control, and blood potassium levels are so high that they can cause cardiac arrhythmias and death. The patient has already lost a lot of weight and cannot eat well. You experience nausea and vomiting, especially in the morning. You get tired easily and anaemia, if not already being treated, is usually at dangerous levels.

When ultrasound of the kidneys is performed, they are usually already atrophied, with reduced sizes. Some patients manage to reach stage V with a few signs and symptoms. Despite little symptomatology, they show numerous laboratory alterations. The longer the start of dialysis is delayed; the worse will be the bone, cardiac lesions, malnutrition, and the risk of malignant arrhythmias. Often, the first and only symptom of end-stage renal failure is sudden death.

Kidney Diseases—Causes, Symptoms, Diagnosis, and Treatment
Kidney disease is a collection of various diseases that attack this organ. Their common denominator is a serious threat to health and life and difficulty in diagnosis in the first phase. What else is worth knowing about them?

Kidney Disease—Causes
It is difficult to identify only one cause of kidney disease because it depends on the patient we are dealing with. However, it cannot be denied that one of the most serious negligence is the patient. Some illnesses result from untreated infections, bacteria cause others, and others are the result of a lack of concern for the kidneys in everyday life. Of course, the causes of kidney disease are not always known to us. Sometimes we can only guess at them, and sometimes they are caused by an inappropriate response from the immune system, and doctors have no idea how to change the way it works. It also happens that problems with the kidneys are a consequence of improper intimate hygiene, which women should be especially aware of.

Kidney Disease—Threat
Care for the urinary tract should be something obvious to us, regardless of our age and gender, but some groups of people are at greater risk of developing it than others. Reference is made to the particular risk in the context of older people who, due to their age, already have a reduced efficiency characteristic of the immune system. The risk is particularly high in the context of men, especially if they have a problem with prostate enlargement; however, women and people with hypertension are also at risk, regardless of their age. It is also worth monitoring the kidneys' condition, knowing that medications are often taken, especially antibiotics and painkillers.

Kidney Disease—Symptoms
Asking about the symptoms of kidney disease is one of the things that makes doctors embarrassed. This is not only because each disease has a slightly different course, but also because it is characterized by development without any symptoms alarming the patient. Worse still, even when health problems do arise, you cannot be sure that they will be properly diagnosed. The signals sent by the body can be so non-specific that patients are treated for months for a different disease than the one they are struggling with.

However, we were to indicate those signals, the appearance of which should raise our alertness, we should first pay attention to changes in the urine. We usually see those that affect its smell, but changes can also affect its appearance, colour, and transparency. Other symptoms depend primarily on the disease we are dealing with.

It sometimes happens that the only alarm signal is increased blood pressure, malaise, drowsiness, and headaches. Even symptoms as surprising as peeling of the skin and vomiting can show kidney problems, and sometimes the patient smells the ammonia, not in the urine but the mouth.

Kidney Disease—Diagnosis
Kidney diseases can be difficult to diagnose, so it's no wonder that prevention is of great importance in treating them. Untreated, they can hinder our normal functioning, sometimes making it impossible. Therefore, it is not worth risking the disease, especially since its diagnosis at an early stage does not have to be difficult. This goal can be achieved with a general urine test. Your GP should issue a referral for them, but you should not give up the examination, even if you do not have time to go for the appropriate document. Urine can be tested in almost any analytical laboratory, and because the testing is not complicated, it is also inexpensive.

Usually, the analysis of protein in the urine is analyzed. Still, it is also important for the doctor to determine whether and in what quantity there are white and red blood cells. It is also good to observe the state of the urine yourself so that the power to intervene immediately, as soon as we notice the first disturbing changes.

Kidney Disease—Treatment
The treatment of kidney diseases depends primarily on the disease we are dealing with in a given case. The doctor also considers the general condition of the patient, which is of great importance in the case of older people. Pharmacological treatment is usually of key importance, as it allows to eliminate the symptoms and causes of the disease.

However, the patient is also expected to change the diet, give up stimulants, and take greater care of the quantity and quality of fluids consumed. Unfortunately, while pharmacology is increasingly effective, it is also failing under certain circumstances. In the case of uremia, we are dealing with long-term treatment, which often ends with dialysis, and a patient with kidney cancer must take into account that at some point, removing an infected organ will be the only chance for him to protect himself from death. Many patients benefit from pyelonephritis by having an operation during which a catheter is inserted into the bladder. Systematic medical control is also recommended in each case.

Kidney Disease—Consequences of Neglect
Not all patients decide to treat kidney diseases, even if they are chronic. Therefore, it is worth remembering that the consequence of this approach is usually a renal failure. When it occurs, more and more poisonous substances appear in the patient's body when the blood is not cleaned properly, causing problems with the proper functioning of other organs, including such important ones as the heart, liver, brain, and endocrine glands. In extreme cases, the patient's carelessness leads to the need for dialysis and even a kidney transplant.

CHAPTER THREE:
BENEFITS OF FOLLOWING A RENAL DIET

You need a meal plan that includes a kidney diet if you have a kidney disorder. You will help stay healthy if you notice what you eat and drink. The facts in this section apply to individuals with kidney disease who are not treated with dialysis.

We are all different, and our nutritional needs are different for everyone. Talk to your kidney dietician (a diet and nutrition expert for kidney disease patients) to see which meal scheme works best for you.

Ask your doctor to help find a nutritionist. Private insurance and Medicare policies can help pay for dietary appointments.

As part of the hygienic-dietary measures, nutritional advice should be the first recommendation to the patient. Dietary care has always been considered important in chronic kidney disease (CKD), both as a renoprotective antiproteinuric measure in the predialysis stage, as to prevent overweight and malnutrition in all stages, especially the latter in dialysis patients. The first premise is to guarantee adequate caloric, protein, and mineral support. Never the price to pay for a supposedly adequate diet must be insufficient nutrition. The nutrient recommendations should be adapted to the ideal weight—not real—and corrected for energy expenditure and physical activity of the patient.

Why Is It So Important to Follow a Meal Plan?
The things we were eating and drinking can affect your health. Maintaining a healthy weight and eating a balanced diet low in salt and fat can help control blood pressure. People with diabetes can help control blood sugar levels by choosing very carefully what to eat and drink. Controlling blood pressure and diabetes can help prevent kidney disease from getting worse.

A kidney diet helps prevent damage to the kidneys. The kidney diet limits certain foods and prevents the minerals of those foods from accumulating in the body.

Fundamentals of the Renal Diet
With all meal plans, including the renal diet, it is necessary to track the number of specific nutrients you consume, such as:

- Calories
- Protein
- Grease
- Carbohydrates
- Etc.

To make sure you're getting the right amount of these nutrients, you need to eat and drink the correct portion sizes. All the information you need to track your consumption is a "nutritional information" label.

Use the nutrition information section on meal labels to learn more about the foods you eat. The nutrition information will tell you how much protein, carbohydrates, fat, and sodium are in each serving of that meal. This can help you choose foods rich in the nutrients you need and low in the nutrients you should limit.

When you look at nutrition data, some key areas will give you the information you need:

Calorie
The calories you eat and drink are the source of your body's energy. Protein, carbohydrates, and dietary fats are the products of calories. The calorie required depends on your age, sex, body size, and level of activity.

You can adjust your calorie consumption by weight. Some people restrict their calories; others must eat more calories.

Protein
Protein is one of the body's fundamental components. To grow, heal, and remain healthy, the body needs protein. Skin, hair, and nails could be weakened by too little protein. But there is too much protein. To improve your health and mood, the amount of protein you eat may have to be adjusted.

The number of protein you should consume depends on your body size, level of activity, and health problems. Some doctors recommend people with kidney disease to limit their protein or change their protein source. This is because a high-protein diet can hinder kidney function and cause damage.

Protein intake recommendations vary depending on the stage of the patient. In ACKD, a moderate restriction of protein intake is recommended; in dialysis patients, intakes should be higher to compensate for the catabolic nature of the technique.

Find out which foods are low and high in protein. Remember that just because a meal is low in protein does not mean that you can consume it in high amounts.

Low protein meals	High protein meals
Bread	Red meat
Fruits	Chicken
Vegetables	Fish
Pasta and rice	Eggs

Protein Restriction in ACKD
The kidney is the natural route of elimination of nitrogenous products. It is based on the fact that unlike sugars and fats whose final product is H_2O and CO_2, the final product of protein metabolism is nitrogen, which is eliminated mainly by the kidneys in the form of urea. With renal failure progression, these nitrogenous products (together with phosphates, sulphates, and organic acids) accumulate in proportion to the loss of renal function. This not only gave rise to the principle of protein restriction but also to the urea kinetic model to establish the dialysis dose. Protein restriction has been prevalent for decades (since 1918) and has been the cornerstone of treatment when dialysis did not exist.

Hydration

Hydration in ACKD is discussed in an extensive format elsewhere. For dialysis patients, it is recommended to drink as much liquid as is eliminated with the urine in this period, plus an additional 500–750cc. Regarding the patient's weight, the interdialytic gain should not exceed 4–5% of their dry weight. In PD, the fluid balance is continuous, but the peritoneal ultrafiltration capacity is limited, so a moderate fluid restriction and adjusted to the peritoneal balances are recommended.

Salt Intake

The limitation of saline intake is a classic indication, both in patients with ACKD and renal replacement therapy. It is important to prevent hydro saline retention, an adjunct in controlling blood pressure, and even reduces proteinuria and facilitates the effect of renin-angiotensin axis blockers. We must consider it very important to be able to verify the saline intake objectively to favour the adherence of this prescription. The most affordable method of monitoring saline intake is urinary sodium excretion, and we must emphasize the importance of measuring urinary sodium during routine office visits. Now, is urinary sodium useful as an indicator of salt intake? The answer is not easy to find in the literature, and the information must be sought in the classical books of human physiology. Under normal conditions, faecal sodium excretion is less than 0.5% of the intestinal content of the ion, thanks to its rapid and effective absorption by the intestinal mucosa. Therefore, if we consider that the intestine absorbs almost all of the sodium ingested; urinary sodium elimination is a good reflection of salt intake. Although there is always the risk of inadequate 24-hour urine collection, several studies have highlighted that it is the most practical method to verify salt intake.

Grease

To stay healthy, you need some fat in your food plan. Fat gives you energy and helps you eat certain vitamins. However, too much fat can lead to heart and weight gain. Try to limit your dietary fat and, if possible, select healthier fats.

The healthiest fat or "good" fat is called unsaturated fat. Examples of unsaturated fats include:

- Olive oil
- Peanut oil
- Corn oil

Unsaturated fat can contribute to lower cholesterol levels. Try to eat unsaturated fats if you need to gain weight. Limit unsaturated fats in your food plan if you need to lose weight. Modesty is the key, as always. There may be too many problems with 'good' fat.

Saturated fat, also called "bad" fat, may increase your heart disease risk and cholesterol level. Saturated fat examples contain:

- Butter
- Lard
- Shortening
- Meats

Limit these fats in your eating plan. Choose healthy, unsaturated fats instead. Cutting the amount of fat in meats and removing the skin from chicken or turkey can also limit saturated fat. Trans fats should also be avoided. This kind of fat increases your 'bad' cholesterol and decreases your 'good' cholesterol. If this occurs, your heart disease may be more likely to lead to kidney damage.

Sodium
Sodium (salt) is a mineral found in almost every food. Too much sodium can thirst, which can cause bloating and increase blood pressure. This can damage your kidneys and make it harder for your heart to work.

One of the best ways to stay healthy is to limit your sodium intake. To control the sodium in your meal plan:
- Do not add salt to your food when you are cooking or eating. Try to cook with fresh herbs, lemon juice, or unsalted spices.
- Choose fresh or frozen vegetables from canned vegetables. If you are using canned vegetables, drain and rinse to remove the salt before cooking or eating.
- Avoid processed meats like ham, bacon, hot dogs or chorizo, and lunch meats.
- Eat fresh fruits and vegetables instead of cookies or other salty snacks.
- Avoid canned soups and frozen meals that are high in sodium.
- Avoid foods such as olives and pickles that have been pickled.
- Limit high-sodium condiments such as soya sauce, barbecue sauce, or ketchup.

Important! Important! Be careful with salt substitutes or "lower sodium" foods. A lot of salt substitutes are high in potassium. Too much potassium can be hazardous if you have kidney disease. Work with your dietitian to find foods that are low in sodium and potassium.

Portions
It is a great beginning to choose healthy foods, but eating too much can be an issue. The other component of a healthy diet is the control of portions or watching how much you eat.

To control portions:

- On all foods, check the label for nutrition facts and learn the serving size. Most bundles have more than one serving. A 20-ounce bottle of soda, for example, is two and a half servings. With nutrition facts labels, fresh foods, like fruits and vegetables, do not come. Ask your dietician for a list of fresh foods for nutrition and advice on measuring portions correctly.
- Eat slowly and when you are not hungry anymore, stop eating. It takes your stomach approximately 20 minutes to tell your brain that it is already full. You may eat more than you need if you eat too quickly.
- When doing something else, such as watching TV or driving, avoid eating. You do not know how much you have eaten when you are distracted.
- Do not eat from the food package directly. Take a portion of food out, instead, and put the bag or box at a distance.

Controlling portion sizes is important to any meal plan. It is even more important on a kidney diet because you may need to limit how much you eat or drink.

What Is the Difference Between Kidney Diets?

Waste and fluids build up in your body when your kidneys are not working as well as they should. This additional fluid and waste can cause heart, bone, and other health problems over time. A kidney diet meal plan can restrict the number of certain minerals and fluids you consume. This can avoid building up and causing problems with waste and extra fluids.

Depending on your stage of kidney disease, it will depend on how strict you must be with your plan. There may be little or no limit to what you eat or drink in the early stages of kidney disease. As time goes by and your kidney disease gets worse, your doctor may recommend limiting:

- Potassium
- The match
- Liquids

Potassium

Potassium is a mineral that is present in nearly all foods. For your muscles to work, your body needs some level of potassium, but too much potassium can be hazardous. Your potassium level can be very high or very low when your kidneys are not working well. Muscle cramps, problems with how your heartbeats, and muscle weakness can be caused by having too much or not enough potassium. You can restrict how much potassium you eat if you have kidney disease. Ask your doctor or nutritionist if you should limit your consumption of potassium.

Find out which foods contain high and low potassium levels. Your nutritionist can help you understand how healthy it is to eat small amounts of your favourite high-potassium foods.

Eat this (Low potassium foods)	Instead of (Foods high in potassium)
Apples, grapes, strawberries, pineapple, and ploughing,	Avocados (avocado), bananas, melons, oranges, plums. and raisins.
Cauliflower, onions, bell peppers, radishes, summer squash, and lettuce	Artichokes, pumpkin, bananas, spinach, potatoes. and tomatoes.
Pita, tortillas, and white bread,	Bran and granola products.
Beef, chicken, and white rice,	Beans, brown or wild rice (baked, black, pinto, etc.)

Match

Phosphorus has been found in nearly all foods as a mineral. Works to maintain your bones healthy, using calcium and vitamin D. Healthy kidneys keep phosphorus in the body at the right level. Phosphorus can build up if your kidneys do not work well. In your blood, too much phosphorus can easily cause bones to break.

There must be phosphorus limits for many people with renal diseases. Please ask your doctor if phosphorus should be restricted. Your doctor may prescribe a medicine called a phosphorus binder, depending on your stage of kidney disease.

This can prevent your blood from developing phosphorus. You may have to look at the amount of phosphorus that you are eating in your diet. To get an idea of how to make healthy choices if you need to limit phosphorus in your diet, use the table below

Eat this (Low phosphorus meals)	Instead of this (Foods high in phosphorus)
Italian, French, or sourdough bread.	Whole grain bread.
Corn or rice cereals and cream of wheat.	Bran and oat cereals.
Unsalted popcorn.	Dried fruits and sunflower seeds.
Light-colour soda or lemonade.	Dark colour sodas.

Our bodies need survival water, but you may not need water so much if you have kidney disease. This is why they do not remove extra fluids as they should if their kidneys are damaged. Too many fluids can be dangerous in your body. High blood pressure, heart failure, and swelling can occur. The additional fluids that you collect near your lungs can make breathing difficult. Your doctor may request that you limit the number of fluids you drink, depending on the kidney disease stage and your treatment. You will need to limit how much you take if your doctor asks you to do this. Some foods containing water will also have to be cut off. Soups and foods melting have plenty of water, like icing cream and gelatine. In water, too, a lot of fruit and vegetables are high. To control how much you drink, you have to limit fluids, measure the quantities of liquid and drink from small glasses. To prevent thirst, limit the amount of salt. You may feel thirsty sometimes. You can do the following to help alleviate thirst:

- Chew gum.
- Rinse your mouth.
- Suck on an ice cube, mint or hard caramel (remember to choose a sugar-free caramel if you have diabetes).

Special Dietary Concerns
Vitamins
Following a diet plan with a kidney diet may prevent your body from getting enough vitamins and minerals you need. To help you get the right levels of vitamins and minerals, your dietician may suggest a supplement created for people with kidney disease.

Therapists or dieticians may also suggest a special type of vitamin D, folic acid, or iron pill to help prevent some side effects typical of kidney disease, such as bone disease and anaemia.

Regular use of many vitamins may not be healthy for you if you have kidney disease. They may contain much or too little vitamin.

After Diabetic Kidney Meal
Should you have diabetes, you need to control blood sugar levels to prevent damage to the kidneys. A doctor or nutritionist can help you create a meal plan that enables you to control blood sugar levels while limiting sodium, phosphorus, potassium, and water. Diabetes educators can also learn to control blood sugar levels. Ask your doctor to introduce you to a diabetes educator in your area. Private insurance and Medicare can help you pay for reservations with diabetic educators.

CHAPTER FOUR:
HOW TO IMPROVE KIDNEY FUNCTION

One of the most important organs in your body is your kidneys. In regulating your blood, blood volume, blood pressure, and blood pH, they have important functions. In the form of urine, they are also responsible for filtering blood and the excretion of waste. To enhance your overall health, and reduce your chances of getting sick, take great care of your kidneys. Many things can go wrong, but you may be less likely to suffer from things like kidney stones, kidney infections, or failure if you follow a few simple tips.

Eat Healthily
Eat a Balanced Diet
This is one of the main factors in good overall health, and your kidneys are no exception. Avoid fatty and salty foods. Consume lots of fresh fruits and vegetables. If you're not sure how to put together a balanced diet, you can use the food pyramid, which divides foods into different groups.

Public health experts criticized the original food pyramid, and you can now find the newer, revised version. Here, healthy foods are combined with other aspects, such as weight control.

Lower the Amount of Salt in Your Diet
It is very normal for people to consume too much salt or sodium in their diet. Foods high in salt or sodium can be particularly bad for the kidneys. High levels of sodium can lead to high blood pressure.

Over time, high blood pressure can damage your kidneys and make you more susceptible to serious kidney disease.

- Choose fresh rather than pre-packaged foods. As a result, you'll typically consume less sodium.
- If you buy pre-packaged foods, make sure that the packaging says 'no extra salt' or something similar.
- Get in the habit of studying food labels and finding out the sodium content of each food.

Eat "Kidney-Friendly" Foods
Adhering to a balanced and healthy diet should be a priority, but some foods are particularly beneficial for your kidney function. Foods with antioxidants—usually fruits and vegetables—can help boost the overall health of your kidneys. Some of the best vegetables to have on your shopping list are cabbage and cauliflower, berries (especially cranberries), red peppers, and onions.

- Although cranberries are very good food for you, store-bought cranberry juice can be high in sugar.
- Asparagus is especially good for your kidneys.

Drink Healthily
Drink a Lot of Water
Staying hydrated has a beneficial effect on your health. If you are well hydrated, your urine is more diluted and thus supports healthy kidney function. Some doctors recommend eight glasses of water a day, but in some cases, more than this amount is recommended. Water supports the flushing of toxins from the body. Moisturizing the body well with fluid, makes this task for the kidneys and helps regulate body temperature better.

Drink Water Regularly
Drink water frequently throughout the day, and don't just swallow half a litre at a time, twice a day. The kidneys regulate the fluid in your body. They can do their job more easily if you drink small amounts frequently.

Only Drink Alcohol in Moderation
Consuming large amounts of alcohol may have serious negative consequences for the functioning of your kidneys. Filtering harmful substances out of your blood is one of the primary jobs of the kidneys. Alcohol is one of the most dangerous compounds that your kidneys have to deal with. The functioning of your kidneys can be negatively affected by excessive alcohol consumption.

Alcohol dries you out, and that can also harm your kidneys, whereas good hydration positively affects kidney function.

Weight Control and Regular Exercise
Control Your Weight
It is important to maintain a healthy weight. Being overweight can increase your blood pressure, which can put even more strain on your kidneys. Stick to a good diet and exercise regularly to maintain a healthy weight and keep your blood pressure low.

Obesity can also lead to diabetes. Diabetes with high blood pressure is the two main causes of kidney disease.

Train Enough
Active life and exercise have several positive consequences for your health and play an important role in weight management. Exercise is also helpful for blood circulation and mobility. The kidneys are relieved in their task of regulating the blood in the body. Exercising regularly can also help prevent diabetes and stabilize your blood pressure.
This will reduce the stress on your kidneys and lower the risk of kidney disease.

- Suppose you are not used to exercising regularly. In that case, it is important to incorporate these activities into your daily routine so that you can soon see the long-term benefits and improvements in kidney function. Achieving this can be difficult if you are a very busy person or a rather easy-going person, but you should make an effort to find the right path.
- Find a sport or activity that you enjoy. This is probably the best way for someone to enjoy exercise if they're not used to it.
- Training together with friends or your partner can be much funnier and more relaxing if you don't want to join a club or team.

Get a Good Supply of Vitamin D When You Exercise Outdoors
Kidney disease can be related to a vitamin D deficit. Activating vitamin D is one of the kidneys' jobs. By getting vitamin D from the sun, you can reduce the pressure on your kidneys.

- To promote kidney function, you need to be in the sun for at least 15 minutes a day.
- Vitamin D also regulates calcium and phosphorus levels in the body.

The Emergence of Kidney Disease
Understand How the Kidneys Work
You can first read a little and educate yourself. Learn how the kidneys operate and what their functions are. In keeping your blood healthy, the kidneys play a major role and thus enable important nutrient transport in the body. They also protect you against disease and balance the pH. If you think about it, you will realise how important your overall health is to the health and good functioning of the kidneys.

Know-How Kidney Disease Occurs
After you understand the function and importance of healthy kidneys, you can learn a little more about how kidney disease is caused. The two most common triggers are diabetes and high blood pressure. There are numerous other causes, including poisoning or injury and trauma. Kidney disease, for example, can develop after a particularly severe blow to the kidneys. Some pain relievers can cause kidney problems with long-term, regular use. If you are taking these drugs, you should check with your doctor.

Ask Your Parents if There Have Been Other Cases of Kidney Disease in the Family
Kidney disease is often hereditary. If your family is prone to kidney disease, you may be at slightly higher risk. If so, you can seek advice from your doctor so that you can avoid inheritable kidney disease as much as possible.

How to Avoid Dialysis

- Optimized blood pressure always setting below 140/90 mmHg; after consultation with the attending physician, possibly even below. This usually does not work without taking medication.
- **Sufficient fluid intake:** approx. 2 to 2.5 litres per day. Every liquid is included, including coffee, tea and soups.
- **Pay attention to your diet:** a high protein intake puts a strain on the kidneys. Therefore, the diet should be "normalized" for protein, with 0.8 grams of protein per kilogram of body weight and day (approx. 64 grams for 80 kilograms of body weight).
- **Also important:** save table salt, no more than five to six grams a day
- Moderate physical activity with light endurance training, 30 to 60 minutes five times a week.
- **No smoking:** Smoking damages the kidneys!
- If you have diabetes, ensure that your blood sugar is controlled well. Values that are too high damage to the kidney.
- Avoid certain pain medications, such as ibuprofen and diclofenac. If in doubt, ask the kidney specialist (nephrologist).
- As little contrast media (containing iodine) as possible should be used during X-ray examinations.
- Regular checks by the nephrologist.

Steps to Control Chronic Kidney Failure
Seek Treatment for Hypertension
The pressure is now considered the leading cause of chronic renal failure. According to nephrologist Nestor Scho, professor at Unifesp, the increase in blood pressure damages the blood vessels of the kidneys and may cause hypertensive nephropathy. "This way, the organ becomes overloaded, and little by little loses its filtering capacity," he explains. Taking care of hypertension is essential even when it is not the cause of chronic renal failure, as it becomes even more important in the advanced stage of the disease.

Control of Diabetes
"Diabetes is the second leading cause of chronic renal failure," says nephrologist Lucio Roberto Requião Moura of Hospital Israelita Albert Einstein. This is because the disease triggers the so-called diabetic nephropathy, a change in kidney vessels that leads to a protein loss in the urine. Also, diabetes favours atherosclerosis, the formation of plaque fat in the arteries that hinders the filtration work of the kidneys.

Over time, more and more toxic substances are trapped in the body, leading to death. Therefore, one way to detect the problem is to do urine tests to find out if the protein is being eliminated. Those already diagnosed with diabetes need to be more aware of their kidney health.

Watch the Weight
Overweight people (discover your ideal weight) have a higher risk of developing hypertension and diabetes, which is reason enough not to let the scale hand rise, says nephrologist Lucio. Added to this is that obesity alters the way blood reaches the kidneys by the influence of certain hormones, overloading the organ. More so, being overweight is a risk factor for high cholesterol and triglycerides.

Adapt Your Diet
When it comes to food, analysing the underlying disease that triggered kidney failure is critical. If it is diabetes, for example, the diet should be the right diet for those with diabetes. If it is hypertension, then there should be reduced salt intake. "However, in general, it is recommended that the patient avoid excessive protein intake, especially of animal origin, which gives rise to toxic elements in the body that would make the kidneys work harder," explains nephrologist Nestor. In specific cases of insufficiency yet, there may be retention of potassium in the body. Patients with this problem need to prepare food in a way that causes them to release some of this nutrient. Vegetables, for example, need to be cooked.

Inquire About Medications
Self-medication is dangerous even for healthy people. For those with kidney failure, however, use without proper medical evaluation can accelerate kidney deterioration. "The most dangerous are non-hormonal anti-inflammatory drugs," warns nephrologist Lucio. Therefore, explain your problem at the beginning of every medical appointment to avoid aggravating the disease.

Way to Drink Alcohol
Although no studies prove the isolated relationship between alcohol intake and chronic renal failure, alcohol abuse compromises the functioning of the body as a whole. Thus, it is recommended to handle your consumption. However, if you are going to have a drink nephrologist Nestor advises to opt for wine. "It contains antioxidants that can help eliminate concentrated toxins in the body," he says

Put Out the Cigarette
"Cigarettes are responsible for worsening blood pressure levels and are still involved with hormonal changes that worsen kidney function," explains nephrologist Lucio. Also, smoking triggers a vasoconstriction effect, decreasing the volume of blood filtered by the kidneys. In this case, there is no moderation option. The patient must end the addiction.

Practice Exercises
The last recommended care for chronic kidney failure sufferers is regular exercise. "It prevents diabetes, hypertension, obesity, among other problems, and improves circulation and kidney function," says nephrologist Nestor. According to him, any activity is already better than physical inactivity. Still, it is always recommended to seek training that pleases the patient not to feel discouraged over time.

CHAPTER FIVE:
FOODS TO AVOID IF YOU HAVE BAD KIDNEY

The kidneys are the small, bean-like organs responsible for performing some of the most important bodily functions. For example, the kidneys are responsible for generating important hormones, eliminating waste when urinating, filtering the blood, and maintaining a balance of fluids and minerals.

Kidney disease or damage renders the kidneys unfit to perform any of these functions, wreaking havoc on the human body. Several risk factors increase the likelihood of kidney disease, for example, excessive hypertension and uncontrolled diabetes. Some other common causes of kidney disease include heart disease, HIV infection, alcoholism, and hepatitis C.

Once the kidneys become damaged and lose their ability to fulfil their responsibility, an excessive accumulation of fluids, minerals, and waste products begins to accumulate within the bloodstream. However, you can prevent further damage and increase your kidney's ability to function by eating an effective diet that contains foods that do not harm the kidneys and help reduce the accumulation of waste, minerals, and fluids.

Dietary recommendations and restrictions generally depend on the stage of kidney disease or the extent of damage that has occurred and vary according to it. Compared to patients in the late stage of kidney damage or kidney failure, patients who experience the early symptoms of chronic kidney disease will receive markedly different dietary restrictions and recommendations.

Patients who experience late-stage kidney failure symptoms, and are treated with dialysis, a treatment that removes fluid build-up and removes waste products, will receive different dietary recommendations. Most patients suffering from symptoms of late-stage or end-stage renal failure have no choice but to adopt a diet suitable for the kidneys and avoid foods that threaten to create an excessive accumulation of harmful chemicals or nutrients in the bloodstream.

Among patients with chronic kidney disease, the kidneys cannot adequately remove excess phosphorus, potassium, and sodium from the bloodstream. Therefore, these minerals put them at risk for elevated blood levels. An effective kidney diet revolves around consuming foods and beverages that will ensure that your sodium and potassium intake does not exceed 2000 mg per day, while phosphorus intake cannot increase more than 1000 mg per day.

Kidneys that are damaged tend to have a hard time filtering waste products that are made when protein is metabolized. Therefore, patients with stage 1–4 symptoms of chronic kidney disease should reduce their protein intake. However, patients taking dialysis treatment with end-stage renal failure require increased protein intake.

Foods that you must eliminate for an effective kidney diet:

Cola Soda
Calories and sugar are loaded with sugar-filled sodas and artificially flavoured colas, and they also contain a variety of phosphorus-brimming harmful additives, especially dark coloured drinks. Phosphorus is used by most food manufacturers to process food and beverage products, specifically to enhance their taste, increase shelf life, and reduce discolouration. Research shows that artificially added phosphorus, compared to phosphorus consumed by animal meat, plants, or other natural sources, tends to be much more absorbable by the body.

Artificial phosphorus additives tend to have a composition different from natural phosphorus and are therefore not protein-bound. As a type of salt that is easily absorbed from the intestinal tract, these additives are present. In the ingredient list for products, artificially added phosphorous is included, but regulations do not require food manufacturers to specify the exact amount of additive phosphorous added to their product.

The additive phosphor present is highly dependent on the variety you are consuming, but research reveals that most dark coloured glues contain around 50–100mg of additive phosphorus. Therefore, they must be strictly eliminated from an effective kidney diet.

Avocados
Avocados are nutritional superfoods that are considered immensely beneficial and essential due to these rich concentrations of heart-healing antioxidants, fats, and fibre. However, despite being such a healthy staple, they are a dangerous food for people struggling with kidney disease.

This is mainly due to the incredibly rich potassium concentration found in avocados. For example, a 150-grams serving of avocados contains an alarmingly high amount of 727mg of potassium, which is twice the potassium amount present in a medium-sized banana.

Think about it; one cup of avocado can provide you with more than 37% of your daily potassium restriction of 2000mg. Therefore, it is highly recommended to eliminate avocados and avocado-based products, such as guacamole.

Canned Food
Canned foods, including legumes, fruits, vegetables, sauces, and soups, are often brought home due to undeniable convenience and affordability. Many people who commonly buy these canned foods are unfamiliar with the alarmingly high amounts of sodium in these foods.

High amounts of salt are added to varieties of canned food as a preservative to improve flavour and increase the shelf life of the product. Due to the excessively high density of sodium present in most canned foods, it is highly recommended that patients with kidney damage avoid them altogether or limit their portion sizes if they add them to their diets. It is always a healthier option to choose varieties of canned foods that are low in sodium or labelled "no added salt." You can also reduce sodium density by 30–80% simply by rinsing and draining canned foods. This technique works best with canned legumes and tuna.

Wholemeal Bread
Whole wheat bread is widely considered the healthiest option for a perfectly balanced diet, and more refined and processed white flour bread is discouraged due to its lack of essential nutrients. However, when you have kidney disease or damage, it can be difficult to choose the right variety of bread that doesn't aggravate your symptoms.

Even whole wheat bread is a much more nutritious option due to its rich fiber concentration, but kidney-impaired patients are strongly advised to choose white bread over whole grain varieties. You see, whole wheat bread contains a high concentration of potassium and phosphorus, and the higher the concentration of bran and whole grains, the higher the concentration of these two nutrients.

For example, a 30-gram serving of whole wheat bread will provide you with 69mg of potassium and about 57mg of phosphorus. On the other hand, a one-ounce serving of white bread will only provide you with 28mg of potassium and phosphorus. Just keep in mind that most processed bread and packaged bread products, whether whole wheat or white, also contain large amounts of sodium.

It is strongly recommended to select the pieces of bread after comparing and examining the nutrition labels of various varieties. Make sure to choose a variety that is low in sodium, and it's also important to cut down on your portions and limit your intake as much as you can.

Integral Rice
Like whole wheat bread and other products, brown rice is also a whole grain and therefore contains a much higher density of potassium and phosphorus than white rice. For example, a cup of cooked brown rice will provide you with 154mg of potassium and 150mg of phosphorus. On the other hand, a cup of cooked rice will only provide you with 54mg of potassium and 69mg of phosphorus.

You can add brown rice to your diet as long as you can control your portion sizes and eat them occasionally by balancing it with other foods that are low in phosphorus and potassium. It is highly recommended to choose grains that are low in phosphorus, such as buckwheat, couscous and pearl barley, which are much safer alternatives for an effective kidney diet.

Bananas
Bananas are popular for packing an incredibly rich concentration of potassium. Although they naturally contain lower sodium concentrations, a medium-sized banana will give you 422mg of potassium. If you are in the habit of consuming more than two bananas a day, it can be extremely difficult to keep your daily potassium intake below 2000mg.

If you like to eat tropical fruits, be aware that almost all varieties contain extremely rich potassium concentrations. However, pineapples have a considerably lower potassium density compared to other tropical fruits.

Dairy Products
Dairy products contain a rich concentration of nutrients and vitamins; they are an essential part of a healthy and balanced diet. But dairy products are also rich in potassium, phosphorus, and protein, making them a hazardous dietary ingredient for kidney disease patients.

In patients with kidney disease, regular consumption of various dairy products and other foods rich in phosphorus can be hazardous to bone health. This is a surprise because the calcium content is widely recommended for strengthening the muscles and bone structure in dairy products, particularly milk.

Research reveals that excessive phosphorus consumption will lead to a build-up of phosphorus in the bloodstream when the kidneys are diseased or damaged. This will lead to excessive weakness and thinness of the bone structure over time, leading to an increased risk of bone fractures or breaks.

Dairy products also tend to be high in protein. Patients with kidney disease should take steps to reduce their intake of dairy products to prevent excessive build-up of protein residues in the bloodstream. Instead of whole milk, you can choose safer substitutes that contain much lower concentrations of protein, phosphorus, and potassium compared to cow's milk and dairy products. For example, rice milk and almond milk are excellent alternatives to whole milk in the diet of the kidneys.

Oranges and Orange Juice
Even though oranges and freshly squeezed orange juice are among the richest and healthiest sources of vitamin C, these citrusy delicacies also contain an incredibly high concentration of potassium. A large orange can provide you with an alarming 333mg of potassium. But orange juice contains a higher density.

Considering their dangerously high potassium concentration, it is best to avoid oranges and orange juice, and if you must add it to your kidney diet, reduce the portions. Instead of oranges, you can select healthier fruits that contain lower potassium densities, such as grapes, blueberries, and apples.

Processed Meats
A large body of research establishes a direct association between the regular consumption of processed meats and risk factors for chronic diseases. Processed meats are considered one of the least healthy staples because they accumulate an alarmingly high preserves concentration.

Processed meats are canned, dried, salted, or cured meats, for example, sausage, bacon, pepperoni, jerky, etc. Processed meats are packed with dangerously high amounts of salt, which enhance flavour and preserve the flavour for longer shelf life. Additionally, these processed meats also contain a high density of protein. If your doctor has specifically instructed you to reduce your protein intake, consuming processed meats regularly is an unhealthy habit for you.

Pickles, Olives, and Sauce
Pickles, seasonings, and processed olives are the most commonly consumed types of cured or pickled foods. The pickling and curing process involves the addition of unusually large and unhealthy amounts of salts.

Processed olives that are fermented and cured to make their tasteless bitter are also dipped in salt to alter the bitter taste. Five green pickled olives contain an alarming 195mg of sodium, which turns out to be a dangerous serving of sodium in such a small serving. Most supermarkets and grocery stores offer low-sodium varieties of olives, seasonings, and pickles that tend to pack less salt than their traditional counterparts. However, keep in mind that even low sodium varieties tend to accumulate large amounts of sodium. Therefore, it is best to restrict your consumption of processed olives, pickles, and condiments, and if you have to consume them, consume very small amounts.

Apricots
Apricots are a powerful superfood as they pack an incredibly rich concentration of various essential nutrients and minerals; including fibre, vitamin A, and vitamin C. Unfortunately for patients with kidney damage; they also contain dangerously high amounts of potassium. Just one cup of raw apricots contains a whopping 427mg of potassium.

When apricots are dried, their potassium content becomes more concentrated and strengthened. A one-cup serving of dried apricots contains more than 1,500mg of potassium.

It is important to eliminate apricots, particularly dried apricots, to enjoy effective results from a successful kidney diet.

Potatoes and Sweet Potatoes
Even though sweet potatoes and potatoes are not unhealthy vegetables, they can be harmful to a kidney-damaged patient due to their incredibly rich potassium concentration. Consuming a medium-sized baked potato will provide you with 610mg of potassium, while a small-sized baked potato contains 541mg of potassium.

Fortunately, we can reduce the potassium density of several potassium-filled vegetables and fruits, including sweet potatoes and potatoes, simply by soaking or leaching them. Cutting the potatoes or sweet potatoes into small pieces like cubes and boiling them for at least 10–15 minutes will reduce the potassium concentration by 50%.

Another impressive method to reduce potassium content is to put potatoes in a large pot of water for more than four hours before baking or cooking. It causes a noticeable reduction in potassium content compared to potatoes that are not soaked before cooking. This technique is known as potassium leaching and is more popularly known as the double cooking method.

Just be sure to note that while the potassium leaching method helps reduce the potassium content in potatoes, this technique does not remove the potassium completely. Even twice-cooked potatoes and boiled sweet potatoes pack up significant amounts of potassium content. Therefore, it is highly recommended to consume moderately conscious portions so that your potassium levels remain under control.

Tomatoes
Despite containing a beneficial concentration of several essential nutrients, tomatoes are another vegetable loaded with a dangerously high concentration of potassium, so they are not a favourite ingredient for an effective kidney diet. Tomatoes are commonly added to sauces and meals and are also served raw in salads or sandwiches and stewed in soups. Be careful about consuming tomatoes, as just one cup of tomato sauce can contain more than 900mg of potassium.

You can easily alternate tomatoes with roasted red bell peppers to create a flavorful red sauce that will provide you with various nutrients and a considerably lower potassium density.

Packaged, Instant, and Prepared Meals

Processed, ready-to-eat foods and all packaged varieties are major sources of excessive amounts of sodium in our daily diet. These prepared and packaged meals contain excessive salt amounts with no trace nutrients and are best eliminated from a kidney diet.

Most varieties of packaged and ready-made meals typically contain highly processed ingredients and are therefore full of sodium. Some popular consumer varieties include microwaveable meals, frozen pizzas, and packets of instant noodles. In addition to being high in sodium, these processed foods are loaded with unhealthy fats and lack essential body needs.

Swiss Chard, Spinach, and Beet Greens

One of the healthiest green leafy vegetables, containing incredibly high concentrations of nutrients and minerals, particularly potassium, is spinach, beet greens, and Swiss chard. They deliver a potassium concentration that ranges from 140–290mg in a one-cup serving when consumed raw. However, their potassium content increases when these leafy vegetables are cooked, even though their size is reduced.

As long as you're eating moderately portion-conscious, it's okay to add raw spinach, green beets, and Swiss chard to your salads, and avoid cooked meals of these leafy greens altogether to avoid a potassium overdose.

Dates, Raisins, and Plums

Prunes, raisins, and dates are the most widely consumed dried fruits and are popularly added to many packaged baked goods and desserts. Research reveals that when fruits are allowed to dry, all of their nutrients, including their potassium concentration, are converted to a concentrated form.

For example, a one-cup serving of plums contains 1,274mg of potassium, approximately five times the potassium concentration supplied by a cup of raw plums. Even worse is the potassium density of dates, which accumulate a whopping 668mg of potassium with just four dates.

Increasing your potassium intake is dangerous for patients suffering from kidney damage. It is highly recommended to eliminate or at least reduce your potassium intake to enjoy effective results from your kidney diet. Plums, dates, and raisins simply cannot be included on the list due to their dangerously high potassium concentration.

Pretzels, Chips, and Cookies

Crackers, potato chips, and pretzels are very low in nutrients and contain dangerously unhealthy salt amounts. Besides, it is very easy to consume large amounts of these foods, causing you to consume much more salt than you intend to consume. Patients with kidney disease should reduce their intake of phosphorus, potassium, and sodium, as their reduction is strongly related to the reduction and management of symptoms.

Due to the absence of goodies on the menu, it can be extremely difficult to go on a kidney diet, making eating very restrictive and disappointing. However, foods that contain dangerously high amounts of phosphorus, sodium, and potassium should be avoided. For assistance in designing a diet plan specific to your kidney condition, be sure to consult your renal specialist, nutritionist, or dietitian. The dietary restrictions and suggestions you should follow will naturally depend on the severity of your symptoms and the extent to which your body has suffered kidney damage.

Best Foods for People with Kidney Disease

Restrictions in diet depend a lot on the degree of kidney damage. Generally, to protect these organs, we ask to limit the consumption of sodium, the main component of salt, potassium and phosphorus. Proteins should also be wary of, as their waste products can strain the kidneys.

Here are the best foods for people with kidney disease.

1. **Cauliflowers:** Cauliflower has many benefits. They contain fibre, vitamins C, K, and the B group. They are also anti-inflammatory and can be used in place of potatoes.

One cup of cooked cauliflower contains:
- **Sodium:** 19mg
- **Potassium:** 176mg
- **Phosphorus:** 40mg

2. **Blueberries:** Blueberries are a treasure trove of well-being. In particular, they contain antioxidants, such as anthocyanins, which protect us from cardiovascular disease, certain types of cancer, cognitive decline, and diabetes.

One cup of blueberries contains:
- **Sodium:** 1.5mg
- **Potassium:** 114mg
- **Phosphorus:** 18mg

3. **Sea bass:** Bass contains high-quality protein and valuable Omega 3s, which help reduce inflammation and can help counter the risk of cognitive decline, depression, and anxiety. Unlike many other fish that are rich in phosphorus, sea bass has little of it.

One hundred grams of cooked sea bass contain:
- **Sodium:** 80mg
- **Potassium:** 290mg
- **Phosphorus:** 230mg

4. **Black grapes:** Grapes are full of vitamin C and antioxidants capable of reducing inflammation. Furthermore, the berries are particularly rich in resveratrol, a precious flavonoid that helps the heart and brain.

Half a cup of black grapes contains:
- **Sodium:** 1.5mg
- **Potassium:** 144mg
- **Phosphorus:** 15mg

5. Egg whites: Although egg yolks are very nutritious, they contain high amounts of phosphorus, which is not beneficial to those with delicate kidneys. Egg whites, on the other hand, are an excellent choice.

Two egg whites contain:
- **Sodium:** 110mg
- **Potassium:** 108mg
- **Phosphorus:** 10mg

6. Garlic: They can be a tasty alternative to the use of salt. They also contain a good dose of manganese, vitamins C and B6, and contain molecules with anti-inflammatory properties.

Three cloves of garlic contain:
- **Sodium:** 1.5mg
- **Potassium:** 36mg
- **Phosphorus:** 14mg

7. Buckwheat: Grains very often contain a lot of phosphorus, but buckwheat is an exception. It contains B vitamins, magnesium, iron, and fibre. Since it does not contain gluten, it is also ideal for those who have celiac disease.

Half a cup of buckwheat contains:
- **Sodium:** 3.5mg
- **Potassium:** 74mg
- **Phosphorus:** 59mg

8. Extra virgin olive oil: It is healthy and phosphorus-free.

30 grams of olive oil contain:
- **Sodium:** 0.6mg
- **Potassium:** 0.3mg
- **Phosphorus:** 0mg

9. Broken wheat: Known as bulgur, cracked wheat is an ancient kidney-friendly grain. It is a good strong in B vitamins, magnesium, iron, and manganese. It also contains fibre and protein.

One hundred grams of bulgur contains:
- **Sodium:** 4.5mg
- **Potassium:** 62mg
- **Phosphorus:** 36mg

10. **Cabbage:** The cabbage belongs to a cruciferous cauliflower-like tree. It is rich in antioxidants, minerals, and vitamins.

One cup of cooked cabbage contains:
- **Sodium:** 13mg
- **Potassium:** 119mg
- **Phosphorus:** 18mg

11. **Skinless chicken:** Chicken is kidney-friendly if cooked and then eaten skinless. We never try to buy cooked chicken because it is enriched with sodium and phosphorus.

One hundred grams of skinless chicken contains:
- **Sodium:** 70mg
- **Potassium:** 230mg
- **Phosphorus:** 200mg

12. **Peppers:** Peppers contain an impressive amount of nutrients and little potassium, unlike many vegetables. They are rich in vitamin C; they also contain vitamin A.

A small pepper contains:
- **Sodium:** 3mg
- **Potassium:** 156mg
- **Phosphorus:** 19mg

13. **Onions:** They are also an excellent trick to give flavour to foods using a little salt and, therefore, sodium. Besides, onions are rich in vitamins C and B, manganese, and fibre.

A small onion contains:
- **Sodium:** 3mg
- **Potassium:** 102mg
- **Phosphorus:** 20mg

14. **Rocket salad:** It is a salad with a lot of flavours and many benefits. It is rich in vitamin K, manganese, and calcium. It also contains nitrates, which help lower blood pressure.

One cup of rocket contains:
- **Sodium:** 6mg
- **Potassium:** 74mg
- **Phosphorus:** 10mg

15. **Macadamia nuts:** Nuts are high in phosphorus. Macadamia nuts are not, as well as being rich in healthy fats, B vitamins, magnesium, copper, iron, and manganese.

30 grams of macadamia nuts contain:
- **Sodium:** 1.4mg
- **Potassium:** 103mg
- **Phosphorus:** 53mg

16. **Radishes:** They have little potassium and phosphorus, unlike vegetables in general. They are also rich in vitamin C and antioxidants. Their spicy flavour helps to use even less salt.

Half a cup of radishes contains:
- **Sodium:** 23mg
- **Potassium:** 135mg
- **Phosphorus:** 12mg

17. **Turnips:** It has vitamins C, B6, manganese, and calcium; they are perfect allies for the kidneys.

Half a cup of cooked turnips contains:
- **Sodium:** 12.5mg
- **Potassium:** 138mg
- **Phosphorus:** 20mg

18. **Pineapple:** It usually contains a lot of potassium. Pineapple does not. It is also rich in fibre, B vitamins, manganese and bromelain, which reduces inflammation.

One cup of pineapple chunks contains:
- **Sodium:** 2mg
- **Potassium:** 180mg
- **Phosphorus:** 13mg

19. **Redberry:** Cranberries are especially valuable for the urinary tract and kidneys. They contain phytonutrients that make sure that bacteria do not remain in the urinary tract.

One hundred grams of cranberries contain:
- **Sodium:** 2mg
- **Potassium:** 85mg
- **Phosphorus:** 13mg

20. **Shiitake mushrooms:** They are a very tasty ingredient, rich in B vitamins, copper, manganese, and selenium.

One cup of cooked Shiitake contains:
- **Sodium:** 6mg
- **Potassium:** 170mg
- **Phosphorus:** 42mg

Daily Tips to Boost Your Kidney Function
The diet for kidney dialysis helps maintain the balance of electrolytes, minerals, and fluids in dialysis patients. The special diet is important because all waste products are not effectively removed by dialysis alone. Between dialysis treatments, these waste products can also build up.

Most patients with dialysis urinate very little or not, and fluid restriction between treatments is very important. Without urination, fluid in the heart, lungs, and ankles will build up in the body and cause excess fluid.

Dialysis seeks to eliminate the waste of excess water and nitrogen, thereby reducing renal failure symptoms. Dialysis can be used temporarily as a permanent, life-sustaining treatment if the client has acute renal failure or if the client has chronic renal failure. In the latter case, dialysis must continue for the remainder of the patient's life unless successful kidney transplantation is performed.

The kidney dialysis diet is also used in combination with dialysis to control uremia and physically prepare the client to receive a transplanted kidney. Usually, dialysis is necessary until a suitable kidney donor kidney is found to keep the client alive. If the transplanted kidney does not immediately function properly, dialysis may help prevent uremia until the kidney starts functioning properly.

Here are some general guidelines on what to do before or after the commencement of dialysis treatment:

- Eat meals periodically.
- In your diet, include plenty of variety. This will provide you with essential nutrients, such as protein, calories, vitamins, and minerals. They keep you well-nourished with these nutrients.
- Eat some high-fibre foods, such as cereals and whole grain bread.
- Just eat a moderate amount of fat.
- If you have high blood pressure, avoid adding extra salt to your food.

CHAPTER SIX:
DIET FOR CHRONIC KIDNEY DISEASE

Removing waste and purifying the blood is the major role of the kidneys. In addition to this, in removing excess water, minerals, and chemicals, the kidney plays an important role. Therefore, it regulates the balance throughout the body of water and mineral salts such as sodium, potassium, calcium, phosphorus, and bicarbonates. The regulation of water and electrolytes may be disturbed in patients with chronic kidney disease (CKD). This is why the hydro-electrolytic balance can be seriously disrupted by the usual intake of liquids, salt, and potassium. Patients suffering from CKD should adjust their diet according to the doctor and dietitian's recommendations to reduce the work of the kidneys already suffering and avoid disturbances in the fluid and electrolyte balance. For MRCs, there is no fixed regime. Each patient has a diet adapted to his or her clinical condition, the stage of his or her renal failure, and the presence or lack of other health problems. Dietary advice for the same patient should be reviewed and regularly reviewed.

The objectives of diet in case of CKD are:

- Slow chronic renal disease progression, thereby delaying dialysis requirements.
- Reduce the toxicity of excess urea in the blood.
- Maintain optimal nutritional status and prevent weight loss.
- Reduce the risk of fluid and electrolyte imbalance.
- Reduce the risk of cardiovascular disease.

High-Calorie Intake
The details of calorie intake in patients with CKD are as follows:

High-Calorie Intake
For daily activities, the body needs calories to maintain a steady temperature, to grow taller, and to have a healthy body weight. Fat and carbohydrates primarily provide calories. In a CKD patient, the daily calorie requirement is between 35 and 40 kcal/kg of body weight per day. Proteins will be used to compensate for the caloric needs if this caloric intake is not properly ensured. This breakdown of proteins can have adverse effects on the body, such as malnutrition and increased toxic waste production. In patients with CKD, therefore, it is essential to provide an adequate amount of calories. The patient's calorie needs must be calculated according to his ideal weight and not according to his actual weight. The weight, particularly in patients with malnutrition or diabetes, may be lower or higher than the ideal weight.

Carbohydrate
The body's primary source of calories is carbohydrates. They are found in sugar, honey, cakes, candies and drinks, wheat, rice, grains, potatoes, fruits, and vegetables. Diabetics and obese individuals need to decrease their intake of carbohydrates. In grains such as whole wheat, whole rice, and Indian millets such as finger millet (nachni, ragi) sorghum, bajra, or pearl millet, which also contain fibres, it is best to use complex or slow carbohydrates. A large proportion of carbohydrates, associated with a small amount of simple or fast carbohydrates such as sugar and should not exceed 20 per cent of the total intake of carbohydrates, should constitute complex carbohydrates.

Lipids
Fat provides twice as much energy as carbohydrates or protein and is an important source of calories for the body. Lipids or unsaturated fatty acids (good lipids) are better than lipids or saturated fatty acids contained in red meat, whole milk, butter, cheese, bacon, poultry, Indian clarified butter or ghee, and coconuts, such as olive oil, peanut oil, rapeseed oil, safflower oil, sunflower oil, fish and nuts. Your saturated fat and cholesterol intake needs to be reduced because they can lead to heart disease and kidney damage. The proportions of monounsaturated lipids and polyunsaturated lipids should be paid attention to among unsaturated lipids. It is harmful to have an excessive intake of omega-6 polyunsaturated fatty acids and a high Omega-6/Omega-3 ratio, while the body benefits from a low Omega-6/Omega-3 ratio. Better than pure oil, blends of vegetable oils achieve the goal. Doughnut-based foods, crisps, Vanaspati/Dalda Ghee (palm oil vegetable butter), marketed pastries are potentially harmful and should be avoided.

Protein Restriction
Protein is essential for repairing and maintaining tissue in the body. They also help in the healing of wounds and the fight against infections. Protein restriction reduces the rate of deterioration of kidney function, thus delaying the need for dialysis and kidney transplantation. But excessive protein restrictions should be avoided. Lack of appetite is common with CKD. The combination of protein restriction and lack of appetite can quickly lead to nutritional deficiency, weight loss, lack of strength, and high susceptibility to infections, leading to death. In India, most Indians are vegetarians. Even non-vegetarians don't take animal products every day. The amount of protein is closely linked at the socio-economic level. It remains far from the recommendations of the Indian Council of Medical Research, which recommends 1 gram per kilo of weight per day. Consequently, the protein restriction of 0.8g/kg per day recommended in MRCs to slow its progression is limited. More emphasis should be placed on the quality of the proteins to consume. Attention should be paid to the complex proteins (0.4–0.6g/kg) contained in curdled milk, paneer cheese, soy milk powder, dry soybean pieces and soybeans, white cheese, egg, etc., and for non-vegetarians, egg white or fatty fish of which we can take small qualities.

Water intake
Why Should Patients with CKD Take Precautions Regarding Water Intake?
By removing the excess water in the form of urine, the kidneys play a major role in keeping the body's water supply constant. In CKD patients, urine volume decreases as kidney function deteriorates.

With the appearance of puffiness of the face, edema of the legs and hands, arterial hypertension, the decrease in the volume of urine causes retention and suddenly an excess of fluid in the body. Dyspnea is due to the accumulation of fluids in the lungs. It may kill the patient if these symptoms are not taken care of.

What Are the Signs of Excess Fluids?
Excess water is still called hyperhydration. The most common signs are oedema, ascites (accumulation of fluid in the abdomen), dyspnea, and severe weight gain over a short period.

What Precautions Should Patients with CKD Take to Control Fluid Intake?
To avoid excess or lack of water, take as many fluids as advised by the attending physician. The volume of fluid intake varies from patient to patient and should be calculated based on the urine volume and hydration status of each patient with CKD.

How Many Fluids Are Allowed in Patients with Chronic Kidney Disease?
- In patients without edema and with the correct urine volume, no restriction is advised. But in patients with chronic kidney disease, taking plenty of water to protect the kidneys is a misconception.
- Patients with edema and decreased urinary volume are required to reduce fluid intake. To reduce edema, the number of fluids allowed should be less than the 24-hour urine volume.
- To avoid excess or lack of water, it is advisable to drink the amount of urine increased by 500ml. The 500ml that we add roughly covers the water losses through sweat and breathing.

Why Do Patients with CKD Need to Weigh and Record Themselves Daily?

It is to monitor the state of hydration and early detect an imbalance. Bodyweight remains constant when water intake is made as recommended. Sudden weight gain indicates water overload linked to intake greater than necessary. Weight gain warns patients to reduce their fluid intake. Weight loss usually occurs after diuretic treatment and reduced fluid intake.

Helpful Tips to Reduce Water Intake

Reducing water intake is hard, but these tips can help you do it.

- Weigh yourself at the set time of the day and readjust your water intake according to your weight.
- The doctor will inform you of the number of fluids to take daily. Therefore, we calculate and measure the amount of water drunk every day. Remember that the water intake does not only concern water but also tea, coffee, milk, curds, butter, juices, ice cream, cold drinks, soups including thin dal, etc.
When calculating the volume of water drunk, you will have to take into account the water intake in your diet. Be wary of watermelons, grapes, lettuce, tomatoes, celery, sauces, gelatins, frozen foods such as ice cream, etc., because they are rich in water.
- Cut back on salt, spices, and fried foods in your diet because they increase the feeling of thirst, causing you to consume more fluids.
- Drink only when you are thirsty. Don't be in the habit of drinking or accompanying someone who drinks.
- If you are thirsty, take a small amount of water or try ice cream. Take an ice cube and suck it. Ice stays longer in the mouth than liquids and therefore gives more satisfaction than the same water volume. Remember to count ice cubes as drunk water. To make the calculations easier, you will freeze the required quantity in the ice cube trays.
- To keep the mouth hydrated, you can gargle with water but without swallowing it. Dry mouth can also be combated by chewing gum, sucking on hard candy, lemon wedges, or mint, or using liquid toothpaste to moisturize the mouth.
- Always use a small glass for drinking; this will help you limit your water intake.
- Take your medicine after meals with the water you drink at these times; this will save you additional water to swallow your tablets.
- The patient must attend to work. An unoccupied person often feels the need to drink water.
- Hyperglycemia in diabetics increases the feeling of thirst. It is, therefore, essential to have strict glycemic control.
- During the hot season, thirst increases. It is therefore recommended to live in the comfort of freshness to avoid the thirst.

How do you measure and consume precisely the prescribed daily amount of fluids?

- The exact amount of water prescribed by the attending physician per day should be placed in a container.
- The patient should remember that he or she is not allowed to drink more than the container's contents over and over again throughout the day.
- Each time the patient drinks something else, he must assess the amount and deduct it from the water in his container.
- Once the container has been emptied, the patient should know that he will not drink anything more during the current day. Therefore, it is advisable to distribute the authorized quantity of water throughout the day to avoid adding more.
- This control method should be done every day.
- Thanks to this simple but effective method, the authorized quantity of water per day is respected.

Salt Restriction (Sodium)
Why Do Patients with CKD Need to Take Less Salt?
Dietary Sodium is important for maintaining blood volume and blood pressure. The kidneys play an important role in regulating sodium. In patients with CKD, the kidneys cannot remove excess sodium and water.

Thus, sodium and water are found in excess in these patients. Excess sodium increases thirst, edema, dyspnea, and high blood pressure. To prevent or reduce these problems, patients with CKD should reduce their salt intake.

What Is the Difference Between Salt and Sodium?
The words salt and sodium are often used synonymously. The salt that everyone knows is sodium chloride, which contains 40% sodium. Salt is the main source but not the only source of sodium in our diet.

There are a few other sources of sodium in our diet like:

- **Sodium Alginate:** Used in ice creams and milk chocolates.
- **Sodium Bicarbonate:** Used as baking powder and sodas.
- **Sodium Benzoate:** Used as a preservative in sauces.
- **Sodium Citrate:** Used to enhance the taste of gelatin, desserts, and beverages.
- **Sodium Nitrate:** Used in preserving and as a colouring agent in certain dishes.
- **Sodium Saccharide:** Used as a sweetener.
- **Sodium Sulphite:** Used to prevent discolouration of dried fruits.

The compounds mentioned above contain sodium without having a salty taste. The sodium is "hidden" in it.

How Much Salt Should We Take?
The amount of salt ingested by Indians on average is 6 to 8g/day. Patients with CKD should take the amount recommended by their doctor. Patients with CKD with edema and high blood pressure are often required to take around 3g/day.

What Foods Are High in Sodium?
Foods high in sodium are:

- Table salt (salt that everyone knows), yeast.
- Papadum, salted pickles, salted chutney sauces, sauces, mixes for seasoning or chaat masala and sambharas.
- Bakery products like cookies, cakes, pizzas, and bread.
- Foods containing yeast such as certain Indian foods such as ganthiyas, pakoras or vegetable fritters, dhoklas made from fermented rice paste, handvo or Gujarat cake, samosa fritters, ragda patties, dahi vadas, etc.
- Wafers, crisps, popcorn, savory donuts, salted dried fruits such as pistachios, peanuts, canned foods, etc.
- Butter and salted cheeses.
- Instant foods like noodles, spaghetti, macaroni, cornflakes, etc.
- Vegetables such as cabbage, cauliflower, fenugreek, beets, radish, coriander leaves, etc.
- Drinks such as salted lassi, masala soda, lemon lemonade, and coconut water.
- Medicines such as sodium bicarbonate, antacids, and laxatives.
- Foods for non-vegetarians like meat, chicken, animal offal like kidneys, liver, and brains.
- Seafood such as crabs, lobsters, oysters, shrimp and fatty fish such as columbi, kurang, crab, mackerel, and dried fish.

Practical Advice to Reduce Your Salt Intake
- Reduce salt intake and avoid adding salt to dishes made with yeast. Prepare your meals without salt and just add the authorized amount. This is the best way to control the amount of salt ingested per day.
- Do not serve savoury dishes or savoury seasonings at the table, and do not leave table salt on the dining table. Do not add salt to your salads, rice, curds, Indian bread like chapatti, parathas and bhakri, etc.
- Carefully read the contents of dishes sold in stores. Look not just for salt, but for anything that may contain sodium. Read the instructions carefully and look instead for sodium-free or "sodium-free" or low-salt "low sodium" products.
- Beware of the sodium contained in drugs.
- Boil foods high in sodium and discard the cooking water. This can reduce the sodium content.
- To make the diet tasty little salted, we can add garlic, onion, lemon juice, amchur, bay leaves, tamarind paste, vinegar, cinnamon, cardamom, cloves, saffron, green peppers, nutmeg, black pepper, cumin, fennel, poppy seeds, etc.
- Warning! Avoid salt substitutes because they can contain a lot of potassium. This potassium from salt substitutes may elevate the blood potassium level in patients with CKD and be dangerous.
- Do not drink the softened water. In the process of making this water, calcium is replaced by sodium. Water purified by reverse osmosis is less rich in mineral salts, including sodium.
- If you are at a restaurant, choose foods where there is less sodium.

Potassium Restriction
Why Are Patients with CKD Advised to Eat a Low Potassium Diet?
Potassium is important for the body. The body needs it for the proper functioning of muscles and nerves and regularly beating the heart.

Normally, the potassium level is kept constant through a balance between food intake and the elimination of excess by the kidney. This elimination can be disturbed in the event of CKD, which can lead to an increase in the level of potassium in the body (hyperkalemia) between two dialysis sessions. The risk of hyperkalemia is lower with peritoneal dialysis compared to hemodialysis. The risk is different in the two groups because the dialysis is continuous in peritoneal dialysis while it is intermittent in the case of hemodialysis.

Hyperkalemia can cause muscle fatigue and irregular heartbeat, which can be dangerous. If the hyperkalemia is very severe, the heart may stop beating suddenly and cause sudden death. Hyperkalemia can be life threatening without prior manifestations (the silent killer).

To avoid these serious consequences of hyperkalemia, patients with CKD are forced to reduce their potassium intake.

What Is the Normal Level of Potassium in the Blood? At What Rate Is It Considered High?
- The level of potassium in the blood is 3.5 mEq/l to 5.0mEq/l.
- When the potassium level is between 5.0 to 6.0 mEq/l, it requires a diet modification.
- When the potassium level exceeds 6.0 mEq/l, it becomes dangerous and requires intervention to lower it.
- When the potassium level is above 7.0 mEq/l, it can be life-threatening and requires urgent treatment.

Classification of Foods According to Their Potassium Content
To maintain the correct level of potassium in the blood, certain foods should be avoided as prescribed by the doctor. Based on the potassium content of these foods, they are classified into three categories (very high, high and low in potassium).

- **Very high in potassium:** more than 200mg/100g of food.
- **Rich in potassium:** 100 to 200mg/100g of food.
- **Low in potassium:** less than 100mg/100g of food.

Foods very high in potassium:

- **Fruits:** Fresh apricots, amla, bananas, coconut, custard, guava, pomegranate, currant, kiwi, mango, melon, oranges, papaya, peaches, apples, plums, and sapoti.
- **Vegetables:** Amaranth, eggplant, broccoli, pumpkin, cyamopsis, colocasia, coriander, mushrooms, spinach, beans, yams, raw papaya, drumstick, potatoes, tomatoes, and sweet potatoes.
- **Dried fruits:** Almonds, dates, hazelnuts, dried figs, raisins, and walnuts.
- **Cereals:** Wheat, Bajra, or ragi flour.
- **Dried vegetables:** Beans and dried lentils of different colours.
- **Mixed spices:** Cumin seeds, coriander seeds, dried red chilli, and fenugreek seeds.

- **Non-Vegetable Foods:** Fish such as anchovies, mackerel, crabs, and beef, shellfish such as shrimp, lobster.
- **Drinks:** Bournvita, beer, buffalo milk, coconut water, condensed milk, drinking chocolate, fresh fruit juice, soft drinks, rasam soup, soup, cow's milk, and wine.
- **Miscellaneous:** Chocolate, cadbury, chocolate cake, chocolate ice cream, Lona salt (substitute salt), crisps, and tomato sauce.

Foods high in Potassium:

- **Fruits:** Ripe cherries, lime, lychee, watermelon, pear, and grapes.
- **Vegetables:** Bananas, beets, carrots, safflower leaves, bitter gourd, cabbage, celery, cauliflower, okra, green beans, raw mango, onions, radishes, green peas, and sweet corn.
- **Cereals:** Barley, all-purpose flour (maida), millet jowar, wheat-based noodles, and vermicelli, rice flakes (pressed rice, poha).
- **Non-vegetarian dishes:** Cital, hilsa (fish), katla, magur, liver.
- **Drinks:** White cheese.

Foods low in potassium:

- **Fruits:** Pineapple, cherries, lemon, strawberries, raspberries, and apples (rose apple).
- **Vegetables:** Garlic, pumpkin, squash, broad beans, calabash (turiya), cucumber, fenugreek leaves (methi), lettuce, and sweet pepper.
- **Cereals:** Rice, rava, and wheat semolina.
- **Legumes:** Green peas.
- **Non-vegetarian dishes:** Beef, lamb, pork, chicken, and eggs.
- **Drinks:** Coffee, coca-cola, Fanta, lemonade, lemon juice, Limca, Rimzim, and sodas.
- **Miscellaneous:** Cloves, dry ginger, honey, mint leaves, mustard, nutmeg, black pepper, and vinegar.

Practical Tips for Reducing Potassium in the Diet
- Take one fruit per day, preferably low in potassium.
- Take a cup of tea or coffee a day.
- Vegetables rich in potassium should only be taken after reducing potassium (as explained below).
- Avoid coconut water, fruit juices, and foods rich in potassium (list above).
- Among the foods that contain potassium, choose those that contain the least potassium when possible.
- Potassium restriction is necessary not only in patients with CKD on predialysis but also after the initiation of dialysis.

How Do You Reduce the Potassium in Vegetables?
- Peel and cut the vegetable foods into small pieces, wash them with lukewarm running water, and put them in a large bowl.
- Fill the bowl with hot water (4 to 5 times the food volume) and let it soak for at least an hour.
- After soaking the food for 2–3 hours, rinse it 3 times with lukewarm water.
- Boil the vegetables with plenty of water that you throw in at the end.

- Foods thus boiled can be prepared as desired.
- Thus, you can reduce the potassium level in some foods, but not completely. Therefore, it is preferable to avoid foods rich in potassium or to take it in small quantities.
- As these foods lose vitamins during cooking, vitamin supplements will be taken as prescribed.

Special tips for reducing potassium in potatoes:

- Cut the potato into small pieces, thus maximizing the surface of the vegetable in contact with the water.
- It is the temperature of the water used to soak or boil the potatoes that make the difference.
- Using plenty of water for soaking or boiling is beneficial.

The Restrictive Phosphorus Diet
Why Should Patients with CKD Eat a Low Phosphorus Diet?
- Phosphorus is an essential mineral for strong bones in the body. Often, the excess phosphorus supplied by the diet is eliminated in the urine, thus maintaining a balanced phosphorus level.
- Normal blood phosphorus values range from 4.0 to 5.5mg/dl.
- In patients with CKD, excess phosphorus from the diet is not excreted in the urine, and the phosphorus level increases in the blood. The increase in phosphorus in the blood causes a release of calcium from the bones, thus causing their fragility.
- The increase in phosphorus in the blood causes other manifestations such as itching, the fatigue of muscles and bones, bone pain, joint pain. Stiff bones increase the risk of fractures.

What Foods Are Rich in Phosphorus That Should Be Avoided or Reduced?
Foods very rich in phosphorus are:

- **Milk and derived products:** butter, cheese, chocolate, condensed milk, ice cream, milkshake or milkshake, cheese, or paneer.
- **Dried fruits:** cashew nuts, almonds, pistachios, dry coconut, walnut.
- **Cold drinks:** Coke, Fanta, Mazza, Frooti, beer.
- Carrots, colocasia leaves, corn, peanuts, fresh peas, sweet potato
- **Animal proteins:** meat, chicken, fish, and eggs.

High Intake of Vitamins and Fibres
Patients with CKD suffer from inadequate vitamin intake during pre-dialysis due to severe diet, the way food is prepared to get rid of excess potassium, and lack of appetite. Besides, some vitamins, especially those soluble in water such as vitamins B, C and folic acid, etc., are lost during dialysis. To compensate for inadequate intake and increased losses, patients with renal failure often require supplementation with water-soluble vitamins and trace elements. A diet rich in fibre is beneficial in CKD patients. Thus, it is recommended that these patients take a lot of fresh vegetables and fruits, which are rich in fibres and vitamins.

Designing a Daily Diet

For MRC patients, the daily ration of food and liquids is planned by the dietitian in collaboration and according to the advice of nephrologists.

The main principles of the ration concern:
- **Fluid intake (including liquid from food):** water restriction should be done according to the doctor's advice. The weight curve should be plotted daily.
- **Carbohydrates:** to ensure an adequate caloric intake with cereals, the patient can take the sugar or glucose in food, provided he does not have diabetes.
- **Protein:** Milk, grains, meats, and eggs are the main source of protein. CKD patients who are not on dialysis should reduce the protein intake in their ration. It is recommended to take 0.8 grams per pound of body weight per day. Once dialysis is started, patients need more protein (especially those on peritoneal dialysis). One should avoid eating proteins of animal origin such as meat, chicken, and fish, foods that are also rich in potassium and phosphorus. All proteins of animal origin can be harmful to CKD patients.
- **Lipids:** the rate of lipids (fat) in food intake must be reduced, but the total elimination of butter, clarified butter, or ghee, etc., can be dangerous. Generally, oil made from soybeans or peanuts is useful for the body provided that it is taken in limited quantities.
- **Salt:** Most patients are advised to reduce their salt intake. They are asked not to add table salt, eat foods prepared with yeasts or in very small quantities. Salt substitutes should be avoided because they are high in potassium.
- **Kinds of cereal:** rice and derived products such as flattened or poha rice, puffed rice, or kurmura can be eaten. To avoid taking a single type of cereal, we can vary by taking wheat, rice, poha, sorghum, semolina, and all the flours and cornflakes offered on the market. Barley, corn, and barja should be limited.
- **Seasoning sauces:** different sauces can be taken in prescribed amounts and varying to improve the acceptability of meals. As sauces are liquid, the amount of liquid consumed with it should be counted. If possible, use thick sauces rather than liquid ones. The proportion of sauces must be following the medical prescription.
- To reduce potassium in foods, it is important to soak them in hot water thrown away later after washing. Afterwards, they must be boiled and the additional water discarded. Thus, the ingredient is ready for the method of preparation of your choice. As an alternative to rice in sauces, you can take khichdi or dosha.
- **Plants:** Plants with a low potassium level can be taken without restriction. But plants rich in potassium must undergo the potassium extraction process before consumption. To improve the taste, lemon juice can be added.
- **Fruits:** fruits low in potassium like apples, papaya, and raspberries can be eaten once a day. On the day of the dialysis session, the patient can eat a piece of fruit. Fruit juices and water from the coconut should be avoided.
- **Milk and derived products:** 300 to 350ml of milk or its derivatives such as kheer (rice cake), ice cream, curdled milk, mattha can be consumed. Again, to avoid excess fluids, one should limit the amounts of these products.
- **Cold drinks:** Pepsi, Fanta, Frooti should be avoided. Do not take any fruit juice or water from the coconut.
- **Dried fruits:** Dried fruits, peanuts, sesame seeds, fresh or dry coconut should be avoided.

CHAPTER SEVEN:
7-DAY PLAN: WHAT TO EAT TO DETOXIFY YOUR KIDNEYS FAST

Bad diets, environmental pollutants, and drug residues place a strain on the kidneys. What you need is time to regenerate the philtre organs. You should pay attention to how to get to know a way of life with it that is kidney-friendly and have healthy recipes.

Many think of the liver first when it comes to detoxification and relief. That is right. However, in terms of disposing of harmful substances, it is often overlooked that our kidneys also do amazing things and are vital. Using tiny philtres, the so-called nephrons, they clean over 1,000 litres of blood per day.

In doing so, urea, phosphates, toxins, and drug residues are filtered out, urine forms, and the pollutants are flushed out of the body. However, the philtre organs of about eight million Germans are constantly overloaded, and the function of the kidneys is already impaired. Our lifestyle with poor diet, obesity, high blood pressure, and diabetes is the primary cause.

You should keep this in mind when cleaning and detoxifying the kidneys. Foods that contain a lot of these substances should therefore at least be reduced during the 7-day kidney detox.

The ten most important rules are:

- Avoid sausage and red meat.
- No fast food, no ready meals, please prepare everything yourself as much as possible—then you will know what's in it.
- Eat lots of fresh vegetables and fruits.
- Pay attention to fibre every day, not only whole meal bread but also psyllium husks or flaxseed.
- Season only sparingly with salt, preferably with fresh herbs.
- Refrain from alcohol and coffee.
- Largely reduce fat and sugar.
- Drink around two litres of water a day. More is not good for kidney function unless you sweat a lot, then you should drink more to compensate for the loss of fluid. Important: Not in a few large portions, but a small glass now and then throughout the day. This cleanses the kidneys particularly well.
- Freshly squeezed lemon juice is deacidified (has an alkaline effect in the body due to its minerals) and can protect against kidney stones, as studies show. Drinking the juice of a lemon every day is therefore considered prevention for the kidneys, but also generally for detoxification.
- **Also important:** Set your kidney week as stress-free as possible and ensure relaxation. Stress is an often-underestimated "enemy" of the kidneys.

Kidneys Detox Day 1
- **Breakfast:** herbal tea to taste, whole meal bread with low-fat quark, seasoned with freshly ground caraway seeds, paprika, turmeric.
- **Lunch:** Carrot pasta with spring onions and pine nuts. To do this, cook the whole grain ribbon pasta until soft, sauté the carrots and onions in a little safflower oil during the cooking time, then roast the pine nuts and add them. Mix everything on a large platter, season with fresh herbs such as parsley, and pour a few ricotta dabs over the top.
- **Dinner:** oven vegetables. To do this, wash sweet potatoes, bell peppers, onions, garlic, potatoes, aubergines (choose according to your taste), cut into strips, and place on a tray greased with olive oil, bake at 200° C, season with fresh herbs such as rosemary. If that's too dry for you: Season skimmed yoghurt with garlic and fresh dill and use as a dip.
- **In between/snack:**
    - Fruit.
    - Whole grain pastries, such as sesame pretzel, without the salt crumble.
    - Green vegetable smoothie, for example, with kohlrabi and cucumber, water.
    - Juice of one freshly squeezed lemon, diluted with tap water.

Kidneys Clean Day 2
- **Breakfast:** muesli made from oat flakes, some flaxseed, berries, and low-fat yoghurt, herbal tea.
- **Lunch:** pasta salad with sun-dried tomatoes and oranges. To do this, cook pasta such as farfalle or penne al dente, chop the dried tomatoes, and fillet an orange. Serve the tomato strips and orange fillets with a little olive oil, chop the fresh parsley or chervil and season the dressing with it, add fine fruit vinegar to taste, mix with the pasta.
- **Dinner:** tomatoes and cucumbers with mozzarella, flavoured with high-quality olive oil and fresh basil, served with whole grain bread.
- **In between/snack:**
    - Fruit.
    - Whole grain pastries, such as sesame pretzel, without the salt crumble
    - Orange-red smoothie, for example, with berries, orange and carrot, water.
    - Juice of one freshly squeezed lemon, diluted with tap water.

Kidneys Clean Day 3
- **Breakfast:** Whole grain bread with cream cheese made from goat or sheep milk, seasoned with fresh herbs to taste, such as chives.
- **Lunch:** poultry steak with paprika vegetables (red, yellow, and green peppers, onions, some sour cream) and rice.
- **Dinner:** apple crumble. To do this, peel tart apples, cut into slices, and place in a lightly buttered baking dish. Drizzle with the juice of one lemon. From 100 grams of whole meal flour, a handful of oat flakes, 80 grams of brown sugar, and just as much butter, a pinch of cinnamon, knead a crumbly mass and sprinkle it over the apples, bake in the oven at 200° C.
- **In between / snack:**
    - Fruit.
    - Whole grain pastries, such as sesame pretzel, without the salt crumble.

- Green vegetable smoothie, for example with banana, cucumber, green lettuce, rice milk.
- Juice of one freshly squeezed lemon, diluted with tap water.

Kidneys Clean Day 4
- **Breakfast**: muesli with seasonal berries or apples, buckwheat flakes, oat milk.
- **Noon:** Italian bread salad. To do this, cut the ciabatta into slices, divide into bite-sized cubes, rub with a cut clove of garlic and moisten a little olive oil, briefly toast on a baking sheet in the oven. In the meantime, chop the tomatoes, cucumber, and onions for the salad and place in a large bowl. Prepare the vinaigrette from olive oil, balsamic vinegar, and lots of fresh herbs to taste, mix with the vegetables. Let the bread cool down briefly, fold into the salad and enjoy.
- **Dinner:** vegetable soup (minestrone). Prepare vegetable broth from vegetables to taste—beans, zucchini, carrots, fennel, celery—first sauté the vegetables in olive oil, then fill up with a little water; season with bay leaf, basil, and a pinch of salt (no more). Just before cooking, stir in a handful of soup noodles.
- **In between/snack:**
  - Fruit.
  - Whole grain pastries, such as sesame pretzel, without the salt crumble.
  - Smoothie red, roughly with seasonal berries and banana, water.
  - Juice of one freshly squeezed lemon, diluted with tap water.

Kidneys Clean Day 5
- **Breakfast:** scrambled eggs from two eggs, pour over a diced tomato, season with fresh herbs, with whole meal bread.
- **Lunch:** risotto with radicchio. To do this, sauté risotto rice in olive oil, add a finely diced onion and a clove of garlic, fry briefly, pour a little vegetable stock, and cook over low heat. In another pan, sauté the sliced radicchio in olive oil, add a little salt, add a dash of oat cream and add this vegetable mixture to the risotto, fold in slightly; season with fresh rosemary.
- **Evening:** Baked vegetable stew. To do this, put the finely chopped vegetables of your choice in an ovenproof casserole dish with a lid, such as beans, pumpkin, tomatoes, courgettes, peppers, onions, kohlrabi. Add a cup of water, season with a little salt but a lot of herbs, if you like, also some chilli, cover and cook at 180° C for about 30 minutes. Then pour the ricotta flakes over the casserole and enjoy with the whole-wheat baguette.
- **In between/snack:**
  - Fruit.
  - Whole grain pastries, such as sesame pretzel, without the salt crumble.
  - Green smoothie, for example, with lettuce, pineapple, cucumber, and water.
  - Juice of one freshly squeezed lemon, diluted with tap water.

Kidneys Clean Day 6
- **Breakfast:** Muesli made from millet, seasonal fruit, and rice milk.
- **Noon:** Salmon Pasta with lemon and zucchini. To do this, sauté the salmon and zucchini in a little olive oil, add a little sour cream, season with fresh lemon juice and a little salt. Boil the pasta and mix both, grind the pepper over it.
- **Dinner:** sauté fried aubergines, aubergine slices, and onion slices in a little olive oil, flavour with lemon, add cherry tomatoes and capers to taste. Rice or whole grain baguettes go well with it.

- **In between/snack:**
    - Fruit.
    - Whole grain pastries, such as sesame pretzel, without the salt crumble.
    - Green vegetable smoothie, for example, with romaine lettuce, apple, and water.
    - Juice of one freshly squeezed lemon, diluted with tap water.

Kidneys Clean Day 7
- **Breakfast:** whole grain bread with herbal cream cheese.
- **Lunch:** Gnocchi with tomatoes. Make gnocchi yourself from 500-grams of floury, boiled potatoes, press through a sieve or mash, and knead with 125-grams of flour and an egg, season with a pinch of salt, and nutmeg. Shape the potato dough into rolls, cut small slices, press a fork on each piece, put in boiling water. When the gnocchi float up, they are done.
Simply drizzle with a little liquid butter and flavour with fresh sage, or serve with a simple tomato sauce (fresh tomatoes, onion, garlic, a pinch of salt, a teaspoon of honey). Gnocchi is excellent for freezing, so simply make double the amount and store them in the freezer.
- **Dinner:** asparagus with green vinaigrette, peeled green or white asparagus, boil, drain, prepare vinaigrette with olive oil, balsamic vinegar, and fresh herbs as desired with whole meal baguette.
- **In between/snack:**
    - Fruit.
    - Whole grain pastries, such as sesame pretzel, without the salt crumble.
    - Red smoothie, for example with beetroot (cooked), apple, water.
    - Juice of one freshly squeezed lemon, diluted with tap water.

Myths and Facts about Kidney Disease
- **Myth:** All kidney disease is incurable

Reality: No, not at all. Kidney disease is curable if it is diagnosed early, and treatment is given immediately. Often the disease stops its progression or progresses very slowly.

- **Myth:** kidney failure can happen as soon as a kidney fails

Reality: No, kidney failure happens when it affects both kidneys. Often, there are no clinical manifestations with just one kidney, and the values of creatinine and urea are normal in the blood. But if both kidneys are affected, the body accumulates waste, and creatinine and urea in the blood increase, indicating kidney failure.

- **Myth:** In kidney disease, edema means kidney failure.

Reality: No. In some kidney diseases, edema is present while the kidney function is completely normal (e.g., nephrotic syndrome).

- **Myth:** In all patients with renal failure, edema is present.

Reality: No. Edema is present in the majority of patients with renal failure, but not all. Patients with advanced renal failure without edema are rare but exist. Indeed, the absence of edema does not rule out the possibility of renal failure.

- **Myth:** All kidney disease patients should drink plenty of water.

Reality: No. Reduced urinary excretion leads to significant edema in renal disease. It is, therefore, necessary to make a water restriction to maintain a good balance in some patients with certain kidney diseases. However, patients with kidney stones or urinary tract infections and normal kidney function should drink plenty of water.

- **Myth:** I'm fine, so I don't think I have kidney problems.

Reality: Most patients are asymptomatic (they have no symptoms) during the early stages of chronic kidney disease. Only the high biological values of creatinine and urea are the only key arguments at these stages.

- **Myth:** I feel great and better; I don't think I need treatment for my kidney problems yet.

Reality: Many patients with chronic kidney disease feel good with the right treatment and therefore stop their medications and diet. Interrupting medication and not following the regimen can be dangerous. They can lead to rapid deterioration of kidney function, requiring dialysis or transplantation in a much shorter time.

- **Myth:** Dialysis performed once in a patient becomes a permanent necessity.

Reality: No, the time on dialysis needed for a patient depends on the type of kidney failure. Acute renal failure is temporary and reversible. Some patients require the temporary recourse to dialysis, but most often, following medical treatment combined with a few dialysis sessions, the kidney recovers its functions and completely. The delay in starting dialysis for fear that this need is permanent threatens the vital prognosis. Chronic kidney disease progresses irreversibly to kidney failure. At an advanced or terminal stage, the need for lifelong dialysis is essential.

- **Myth:** Dialysis cures kidney failure.

Reality: No, dialysis does not cure kidney failure, but it is an effective, life-saving treatment for patients with kidney failure by ridding their blood of toxic wastes and excess fluids and correcting electrolyte and acid-base disorders. Dialysis plays the role of the kidney that is no longer able to do its job. It allows patients to become asymptomatic and to be in good health despite their severe kidney failure.

- **Myth:** In kidney transplantation, men cannot give to women and vice versa; transplantation is not possible between the two sexes.

Reality: Men and women can donate to the opposite sex since the structure and functions of the kidney are the same in both.

- **Myth:** Kidney donation can affect the health and sexual function of the donor.

Reality: Kidney donation is completely harmless and safe and has no effect on the health of donors or their sexual functions. Donors live normally, get married, and have children.

- **Myth:** If you want a kidney transplant, you can buy it.

Reality: Selling or buying kidneys is a crime. A transplanted kidney from an unrelated living donor has a higher risk of rejection than a kidney from a related one.

- **Myth:** Now, my blood pressure has returned to normal and I no longer need high blood pressure treatment. I feel better when I don't take it so, why am I going to keep taking it?

Reality: Many hypertensive patients stop treatment if blood pressure becomes normal, especially since they no longer have symptoms or are better off without it. But uncontrolled high blood pressure is a silent killer that can lead to long-term complications like heart attacks, kidney failure, and stroke. So, to protect these noble organs of the body, it is essential to take your treatments regularly and to regularly measure your blood pressure even in the absence of symptoms and that you are in good health.

- **Myth:** Only men have kidneys in a pocket between the legs

Reality: In both men and women, the kidneys are located in the back and upper part of the abdomen, and they are the same size and function. What men have in a sac between their legs are reproductive organs or testes.

RENAL DIET COOKBOOK FOR BEGINNER

200+ Delicious and Easy Recipes with Low Sodium, Potassium and Phosphorus. Includes A Carefully Selected 21-Days Meal Plan to Avoid Dialysis

Elizabeth Cook

INTRODUCTION

The renal diet is a diet for people (mostly diabetics, CKD patients and chronic kidney disease patients) who have special needs when it comes to their nutritional intake. Mostly it includes high amounts of proteins, sodium, potassium, calcium, phosphorus and low amounts of phosphorus, sodium, potassium, potassium, proteins, fat and proteins, so that it usually limits the fat content of food and sets the protein to carbohydrate ratio quite high as well. A low sodium renal diet can be achieved by adding potassium, low sodium intake, and adding fiber. Many people struggle with adding extra fiber to the diet, and many times it is treated as an unhealthy factor. But when added to the renal diet, you will soon understand the benefits.

Phosphate: Consumption of phosphate becomes dangerous when kidney failure reaches 80% and goes to the 4th/5th stage of kidney failure. So, it is better to lower your phosphate intake by counting the calories and minerals.

Potassium: After getting diagnosed, if your results show your potassium level is high in the blood, then you should restrict your potassium intake. Baked and fried potatoes are very high in potassium. Leafy greens, fruit juices are high in potassium. You can still enjoy vegetables that are low in potassium.

Sodium: Adding salt is very important in our food, but when you are suffering from kidney problems, you have to omit or minimize your salt intake. Too much sodium intake can trigger high blood pressure and fluid retention in the body. You need to find substitutes that help season your food.

Herbs and spices that are extracted from plants are a good option. Using garlic, pepper, mustard can increase the taste of your food without adding any salt. Avoid artificial "salts" that are low in sodium because they are high in potassium, which is also dangerous for kidney health.

Recipes from this cookbook are simple, delicious, and healthy. You can even use them as an inspiration to experiment and create your renal diet recipes. These samples can also be considered as snacks for you throughout the day.

Below is a list of food/nutrients you should avoid preventing kidney-related problems: Food to avoid Limit/Avoid Alcohol No more than two drinks a day According to The Association of Diabetic Retinopathy, dialysis and kidney transplantation, Alcohol can be safe if consumed in moderation. 1-2 alcoholic beverages a day while dieting is acceptable. Alcohol consumption should be avoided completely if this is unattainable. Milk and milk products No more than two glasses a day As per " The American Heart Association, " milk and milk products including cheese, cheese products and yogurt can be allowed without any accommodations. However, it is recommended to replace them with low-fat dairy products. Vegetables and beans No more than 2 cups a day, except for one serving a day of soy milk or other protein-rich beverages. A kidney diet is not complete without vegetables and beans. " United States National Library of Medicine" specifies that one banana, one apple, a serving of broccoli, and one cup of tomato juice can be substituted with protein-rich food. Grains No more than two servings a day. It is recommended to substitute them with another high protein low-fat food regular, such as poultry or fish. A cup of milk and two saltine crackers are also allowed a day. If you're already used to the renal diet, you can work with the recipes from this cookbook. You can use the guide for more severe and careful renal diet beginners. If you want to live a happy, healthy renal diet, try these simple recipes for a better taste!

CHAPTER 1:

UNDERSTANDING KIDNEY DISEASE

Kidney disease is becoming more prevalent in the United States, and so we need to learn as much about it as we can. The more we educate ourselves, the more we can do to take care of this important bodily system. If you've been diagnosed with chronic kidney disease (CKD), education can empower you to most effectively and purposefully manage the disease. Once you have a full understanding of what chronic kidney disease is, you can begin to take charge of your evolving health needs. Making healthy changes early in the stages of kidney disease will help determine how well you will manage your kidney health. I am here to guide you, every step of the way. Like any new process, it may seem intimidating at first. But this chapter provides the foundation for learning and will help you understand kidney disease as you begin your journey to healthier kidneys.

What Do the Kidneys Do?
Our kidneys are small, but they do powerful things to keep our bodies in balance. They are bean-shaped, about the size of a fist, and are located in the middle of the back, on the left and right sides of the spine, just below the rib cage.

When everything is working properly, the kidneys do many important jobs such as:

- Filter waste materials from the blood
- Remove extra fluid, or water, from the body
- Release hormones that help manage blood pressure
- Stimulate bone marrow to make red blood cells
- Make an active form of vitamin D that promotes strong, healthy bones

What Causes Kidney Disease?
There are many causes of kidney disease, including physical injury or disorders that can damage the kidneys, but the two leading causes of kidney disease are diabetes and high blood pressure. These underlying conditions also put people at risk for developing cardiovascular disease. Early treatment may not only slow down the progression of the disease, but also reduce your risk of developing heart disease or stroke.

Kidney disease can affect anyone, at any age. African Americans, Hispanics, and American Indians are at increased risk for kidney failure, because these groups have a greater prevalence of diabetes and high blood pressure.

When we digest protein, our bodies create waste products. As blood flows through the capillaries, the waste products are filtered through the urine. Substances such as protein and red blood cells are too big to pass through the capillaries and so stay in the blood. All the extra work takes a toll on the kidneys. When kidney disease is detected in the early stages, several treatments may prevent the worsening of the disease.

If kidney disease is detected in the later stages, high amounts of protein in your urine, called macroalbuminuria, can lead to end-stage renal disease. The second leading cause of kidney disease is high blood pressure, also known as hypertension. One in three Americans is at risk for kidney disease because of hypertension. Although there is no cure for hypertension, certain medications, a low-sodium diet, and physical activity can lower blood pressure.

The kidneys help manage blood pressure, but when blood pressure is high, the heart has to work overtime at pumping blood. When the force of blood flow is high, blood vessels start to stretch so the blood can flow more easily. The stretching and scarring weaken the blood vessels throughout the entire body, including the kidneys.

And when the kidneys' blood vessels are injured, they may not remove the waste and extra fluid from the body, creating a dangerous cycle, because the extra fluid in the blood vessels can increase blood pressure even more.

With diabetes, excess blood sugar remains in the bloodstream. The high blood sugar levels can damage the blood vessels in the kidneys and elsewhere in the body. And since high blood pressure is a complication from diabetes, the extra pressure can weaken the walls of the blood vessels, which can lead to a heart attack or stroke.

Other conditions, such as drug abuse and certain autoimmune diseases, can also cause injury to the kidneys. In fact, every drug we put into our body has to pass through the kidneys for filtration.

An autoimmune disease is one in which the immune system, designed to protect the body from illness, sees the body as an invader and attacks its own systems, including the kidneys. Some forms of lupus, for example, attack the kidneys. Another autoimmune disease that can lead to kidney failure is Good pasture syndrome, a group of conditions that affect the kidneys and the lungs. The damage to the kidneys from autoimmune diseases can lead to chronic kidney disease and kidney failure.

Treatment Plans for Chronic Kidney Disease (CKD)
The best way to manage CKD is to be an active participant in your treatment program, regardless of your stage of renal disease. Proper treatment involves a combination of working with a healthcare team, adhering to a renal diet, and making healthy lifestyle decisions. These can all have a profoundly positive effect on your kidney disease—especially watching how you eat.

Working with your healthcare team. When you have kidney disease, working in partnership with your healthcare team can be extremely important in your treatment program as well as being personally empowering. Regularly meeting with your physician or healthcare team can arm you with resources and information that help you make informed decisions regarding your treatment needs, and provide you with a much-needed opportunity to vent, share information, get advice, and receive support in effectively managing this illness.

Adhering to a renal diet. The heart of this book is the renal diet. Sticking to this diet can make a huge difference in your health and vitality. Like any change, following the diet may not be easy at first. Important changes to your diet, particularly early on, can possibly prevent the need for dialysis.

These changes include limiting salt, eating a low-protein diet, reducing fat intake, and getting enough calories if you need to lose weight. Be honest with yourself first and foremost—learn what you need, and consider your personal goals and obstacles. Start by making small changes. It is okay to have some slip-ups—we all do. With guidance and support, these small changes will become habits of your promising new lifestyle. In no time, you will begin taking control of your diet and health.

Making healthy lifestyle decisions. Lifestyle choices play a crucial part in our health, especially when it comes to helping regulate kidney disease. Lifestyle choices such as allotting time for physical activity, getting enough sleep, managing weight, reducing stress, and limiting smoking and alcohol will help you take control of your overall health, making it easier to manage your kidney disease. Follow this simple formula: Keep toxins out of your body as much as you can, and build up your immune system with a good balance of exercise, relaxation, and sleep.

CHAPTER 2:

THE CAUSES OF RENAL FAILURE

Renal disease, according to experts, requires early diagnosis and targeted treatment to prevent or delay both a condition of acute or chronic renal failure and the appearance of cardiovascular complications to which it is often associated.

In fact, hypertension and diabetes, not adequately controlled by drug therapy, prostatic hypertrophy, kidney stones or bulky tumors can promote onset as they reduce the normal flow of urine, increase the pressure inside the kidneys and limit functionality. Or the kidney damage can be determined by inflammatory processes (pyelonephritis, glomerulonephritis) or by the formation of cysts inside the kidneys (polycystic kidney disease) or by the chronic use of some drugs, alcohol and drugs consumed in excess.

A fundamental role in alleviating the work of the already compromised kidneys is carried out by the diet which is, therefore, the first prevention. It must be studied with an expert nutritionist or a nephrologist in order to maintain or reach an ideal weight on the one hand and on the other to reduce the intake of sodium (salt), and the consequent control of blood pressure, and / or other substances (minerals), without creating malnutrition or nutritional deficiencies. Particular attention should also be paid to cholesterol, triglycerides and blood sugar levels.

Understanding what causes kidney failure goes a long way to deciding just what kind of treatment you should focus on. The most important factor that you should focus on is, of course, your diet. But as you focus on your diet, make sure that you are following your doctor's instructions, in the event of other complications. Let us look at a few of the common causes of kidney diseases.

Diabetes
We do know that diabetes is one of the leading causes of CKD. But we have yet to understand in detail why and how it can cause so much harm to the kidneys.

Time for a crash course in diabetes. What many may already know is that diabetes affects our body's insulin production rate. But what many may not know is the extent of damage that diabetes can cause to the kidneys.

High Blood Pressure
An important thing to remember here is that high blood pressure can be both a cause and symptom of CKD, similar to the case of diabetes. So, what exactly is blood pressure? People often throw the term around, but they are unable to pinpoint exactly what happens when the pressure in the blood increases.

Autoimmune Diseases
IgA nephropathy and lupus are two examples of autoimmune diseases that can lead to kidney diseases. But just what exactly are autoimmune diseases?

They are conditions where your immune system perceives your body as a threat and begins to attack it. We all know that the immune system is like the defense force of our body. It is responsible for guiding the soldiers of our body, known as white blood cells, or WBCs. The immune system is responsible for fighting against foreign materials, such as viruses and bacteria. When the system senses these foreign bodies, various fighter cells, including the WBCs, are deployed in order to combat the threat.

Typically, your immune system is a self-learning system. This means that it is capable of understanding the threat and memorizing its features, behaviors, and attack patterns. This is an important capability of the immune system since it allows the system to differentiate between our own cells and foreign cells. But when you have an autoimmune disease, your immune system suddenly considers certain parts of your body, such as your skin or joints, as foreign. It then proceeds to create antibodies that begin to

Symptoms of kidney disease?
If kidney disease progresses, then the blood level of end products of metabolism increases; this in turn, is the cause of feeling unwell. Various health problems may occur, such as high blood pressure, anemia (anemia), bone disease, premature cardiovascular calcification, discoloration, and change in the composition and volume of urine.

As the disease progresses, the main symptoms can be:

- Weakness, a feeling of weakness
- Trouble sleeping
- Lack of appetite
- Dry skin, itchy skin
- Muscle cramps especially at night
- Swelling in the legs
- Swelling around the eyes, especially in the morning

Diagnose With Kidney Disease
There are two simple tests that your family doctor can prescribe to diagnose kidney disease.

Blood test: glomerular filtration rate (GFR) and serum creatinine level. Creatinine is one of those end products of protein metabolism, the level of which in the blood depends on age, gender, muscle mass, nutrition, physical activity, the foods taken before taking the sample (for example, a lot of meat was eaten), and some drugs.

Creatinine is removed from the body through the kidneys, and if the work of the kidneys slows down, the level of creatinine in the blood plasma increases. Determining the level of creatinine alone is not sufficient for the diagnosis of chronic kidney disease since its value begins to exceed the upper limit of the norm only when GFR is decreased by half. GFR is calculated using a formula that includes four parameters which are; the creatinine reading, age, gender, and race of the patient. GFR shows the level at which the kidneys can filter. In the case of chronic kidney disease, the GFR indicator indicates the stage of the severity of kidney disease.

Urine analysis: the content of albumin in the urine is determined; also, the values of albumin and creatinine in the urine are determined by each other. Albumin is a protein in the urine that usually enters the urine in minimal quantities. Even a small increase in the level of albumin in the urine in some people may be an early sign of incipient kidney disease, especially in those with diabetes and high blood pressure. In the case of normal kidney function, albumin in the urine should not be more than 3 mg/mmol (or 30 mg/g). If albumin excretion increases even more, then it already speaks of kidney disease.

CHAPTER 3:

WHAT YOU CAN EAT, WHAT TO AVOID

Foods You Need
There are many foods that work well within the renal diet, and once you see the available variety, it will not seem as restrictive or difficult to follow. The key is focusing on the foods with a high level of nutrients, which make it easier for the kidneys to process waste by not adding too much that the body needs to discard. Balance is a major factor in maintaining and improving long-term renal function.

Garlic
Excellent, vitamin-rich food for the immune system, garlic is a tasty substitute for salt in a variety of dishes. It acts as a significant source of vitamin C and B6, while aiding the kidneys in ridding the body of unwanted toxins. It's a great, healthy way to add flavor to skillet meals, pasta, soups, and stews.

Berries
All berries are considered a good renal diet food due to their high level of fiber, antioxidants, and delicious taste, making them an easy option to include as a light snack or as an ingredient in smoothies, salads, and light desserts. Just one handful of blueberries can provide almost one day's vitamin C requirement, as well as a boost of fiber, which is good for weight loss and maintenance.

Bell Peppers
Flavorful and easy to enjoy both raw and cooked, bell peppers offer a good source of vitamin C, vitamin A, and fiber. Along with other kidney-friendly foods, they make the detoxification process much easier while boosting your body's nutrient level to prevent further health conditions and reduce existing deficiencies.

Onions
This nutritious and tasty vegetable is excellent as a companion to garlic in many dishes, or on its own. Like garlic, onions can provide flavor as an alternative to salt, and provides a good source of vitamin C, vitamin B, manganese, and fiber, as well. Adding just one quarter or half an onion is often enough for most meals, because of its strong, pungent flavor.

Macadamia Nuts
If you enjoy nuts and seeds as snacks, you may soon learn that many contain high amounts of phosphorus and should be avoided or limited as much as possible. Fortunately, macadamia nuts are an easier option to digest and process, as they contain much lower amounts of phosphorus and make an excellent substitute for other nuts. They are a good source of other nutrients, as well, such as vitamin B, copper, manganese, iron, and healthy fats.

Pineapple
Unlike other fruits that are high in potassium, pineapple is an option that can be enjoyed more often than bananas and kiwis. Citrus fruits are generally high in potassium as well, so if you find yourself craving an orange or grapefruit, choose pineapple instead. In addition to providing high levels of vitamin B and fiber, pineapples can reduce inflammation thanks to an enzyme called bromelain.

Mushrooms
In general, mushrooms are a safe, healthy option for the renal diet, especially the shiitake variety, which are high in nutrients such as selenium, vitamin B, and manganese. They contain a moderate amount of plant-based protein, which is easier for your body to digest and use than animal proteins. Shiitake and Portobello mushrooms are often used in vegan diets as a meat substitute, due to their texture and pleasant flavor.

Foods you Need to Avoid
Eating restrictions might be different depending upon your level of kidney disease. If you are in the early stages of kidney disease, you may have different restrictions as compared to those who are at the end-stage renal disease, or kidney failure. In contrast to this, people with an end-stage renal disease requiring dialysis will face different eating restrictions. Let's discuss some of the foods to avoid while being on the renal diet.

Dark-Colored Colas contain calories, sugar, phosphorus, etc. They contain phosphorus to enhance flavor, increase its life and avoid discoloration. Which can be found in a product's ingredient list. This addition of phosphorus varies depending on the type of cola. Mostly, the dark-colored colas contain 50–100 mg in a 200-ml serving. Therefore, dark colas should be avoided on a renal diet.

Canned Foods including soups, vegetables, and beans, are low in cost but contain high amounts of sodium due to the addition of salt to increase its life. Due to this amount of sodium inclusion in canned goods, it is better that people with kidney disease should avoid consumption. Opt for lower-sodium content with the label "no salt added". One more way is to drain or rinse canned foods, such as canned beans and tuna, which could decrease the sodium content by 33–80%, depending on the product.

Brown Rice is a whole grain containing a higher concentration of potassium and phosphorus than its white rice counterpart. One cup of already cooked brown rice possesses about 150 mg of phosphorus and 154 mg of potassium, whereas, one cup of already cooked white rice has an amount of about 69 mg of phosphorus and 54 mg of potassium. Bulgur, buckwheat, pearled barley and couscous are equally beneficial, low-phosphorus options and might be a good alternative instead of brown rice.

Bananas are high potassium content, low in sodium, and provides 422 mg of potassium per banana. It might disturb your daily balanced potassium intake to 2,000 mg if a banana is a daily staple.

Whole-Wheat Bread may harm individuals with kidney disease. But for healthy individuals, it is recommended over refined, white flour bread. White bread is recommended instead of whole-wheat varieties for individuals with kidney disease just because it has phosphorus and potassium. If you add more bran and whole grains to the bread, then the amount of phosphorus and potassium contents goes higher.

Oranges and Orange Juice are enriched with vitamin C content and potassium. 184 grams provides 333 mg of potassium and 473 mg of potassium in one cup of orange juice. With these calculations, oranges and orange juice must be avoided or used in a limited amount while being on a renal diet.

Some of the high-potassium foods, likewise potatoes and sweet potatoes, could also be soaked or leached to lessen the concentration of potassium contents. Cut them into small and thin pieces and boil those for at least 10 minutes can reduce the potassium content by about 50%. Potatoes that are soaked in a wide pot of water for as low as four hours before cooking could possess even less potassium content than those not soaked before cooking. This is known as "potassium leaching," or the "double cook Direction."

If you are suffering from or living with kidney disease, reducing your potassium, phosphorus and sodium intake is an essential aspect of managing and tackling the disease. The foods with high-potassium, high-sodium, and high-phosphorus content listed above should always be limited or avoided. These restrictions and nutrients intakes may differ depending on the level of damage to your kidneys. Following a renal diet might be a daunting procedure and a restrictive one most of the time. But, working with your physician and nutrition specialist and a renal dietitian can assist you in formulating a renal diet specific to your individual needs.

Renal Diet Shopping List
Vegetables:
- Arugula (raw)
- Alfalfa sprouts
- Bamboo shoots
- Asparagus
- Beans - pinto, wax, fava, green
- Bean sprouts
- Bitter melon (balsam pear)
- Broccoli
- Broad beans (boiled, fresh)
- Cactus
- Cabbage - red, swamp, Napa/ Suey Choy, skunk
- Carrots
- Calabash
- Celery
- Cauliflower
- Chayote
- Celeriac (cooked)
- Collard greens
- Chicory
- Cucumber
- Corn
- Okra
- Onions
- Pepitas
- (Green) Peas
- Peppers
- Radish
- Radicchio

- Seaweed
- Rapini (raw)
- Shallots
- Green lettuce (raw)
- Snow peas
- Dandelion greens (raw)
- Daikon
- Plant Leaves
- Drumstick
- Endive
- Eggplant
- Fennel bulb
- Escarole
- Fiddlehead greens
- Ferns
- Hearts of Palm
- Irish moss
- Hominy
- Jicama, raw
- Leeks
- Kale(raw)
- Mushrooms (raw white)
- Lettuce (raw)
- Mustard greens
- Squash
- Turnip
- Tomatillos (raw)
- Watercress
- Turnip greens
- Wax beans
- Water chestnuts (canned)
- Winter melon
- Wax gourd
- Zucchini (raw)

Fruits:
- Acerola Cherries
- Apple
- Blackberries
- Asian Pear
- Boysenberries
- Blueberries
- Cherries
- Casaba melon

- Clementine
- Chokeberries
- Crabapples
- Cloudberries
- Cranberries (fresh)
- Grapefruit
- Gooseberries
- Pomegranate
- Grapes
- Rambutan
- Quince
- Rhubarb
- Raspberries (fresh or frozen)
- Jujubes
- Golden Berry
- Kumquat
- Jackfruit
- Lingonberries
- Lemon
- Loganberries
- Lime
- Lychees
- Mango
- Mandarin orange
- Peach
- Pineapple
- Pear
- Plum
- Strawberries
- Rose-apple
- Tangerine
- Tangelo
- Watermelon

Fresh Meat, Seafood, and Poultry:
- Chicken
- Beef and Ground Beef
- Goat
- Duck
- Wild Game
- Pork
- Lamb
- Veal
- Turkey

- Fish

Milk, Eggs, and Dairy: Milk:
- Milk (½-1 cup/day)

Non-Dairy Milk:
- Almond Fresh (Original, Unsweetened, Vanilla)
- Almond Breeze (Original, Vanilla, Vanilla Unsweetened, Original Unsweetened)
- Silk True Almond Beverage (Unsweetened Original, Original, Vanilla, Unsweetened Vanilla)
- Good Karma Flax Delight (Vanilla, Original, Unsweetened)
- Rice Dream Rice Drink (Vanilla Classic, Non-Enriched Original Classic)
- Silk Soy Beverage (Original, Vanilla, Unsweetened)
- Natura Organic Fortified Rice Beverage (Original, Vanilla)
- PC Organics Fortified Rice Beverage

Other Dairy Products:
- Non-Hydrogenated Margarine (Salt-Free or Regular)
- Butter (Unsalted or Regular)
- Whipping Cream
- Sour Cream
- Whipped Cream

CHAPTER 4:

MEAL PLAN

Days	Breakfast	Lunch	Dinner
1	Breakfast Salad from Grains and Fruits	Dolmas Wrap	Beef Kabobs with Pepper
2	French toast with Applesauce	Salad al Tonno	One-Pot Beef Roast
3	Bagels Made Healthy	Arlecchino Rice Salad	Cabbage and Beef Fry
4	Cornbread with Southern Twist	Sauteed Chickpea and Lentil Mix	California Pork Chops
5	Grandma's Pancake Special	Crazy Japanese Potato and Beef Croquettes	Caribbean Turkey Curry
6	Pasta with Indian Lentils	Traditional Black Bean Chili	Chicken Fajitas
7	Shrimp Bruschetta	Green Palak Paneer	Chicken Veronique
8	Strawberry Muesli	Cucumber Sandwich	Chicken and Apple Curry
9	Yogurt Bulgur	Pizza Pitas	London Broil
10	Mozzarella Cheese Omelet	Lettuce Wraps with Chicken	Sirloin with Squash and Pineapple
11	Coconut Breakfast Smoothie	Turkey Pinwheels	Slow-Cooked BBQ Beef
12	Easy Turnip Puree	Chicken Tacos	Lemon Sprouts
13	Green lettuce Bacon Breakfast Bake	Tuna Twist	Lemon and Broccoli Platter
14	Healthy Green lettuce Tomato Muffins	Ciabatta Rolls with Chicken Pesto	Chicken Liver Stew
15	Chicken Egg Breakfast Muffins	Marinated Shrimp Pasta Salad	Simple Lamb Chops
16	Breakfast Egg Salad	Peanut Butter and Jelly Grilled Sandwich	Chicken and Mushroom Stew

17	Vegetable Tofu Scramble	Grilled Onion and Pepper Jack Grilled Cheese Sandwich	Roasted Carrot Soup
18	Cheese Coconut Pancakes	Crispy Lemon Chicken	Garlic and Butter-Flavored Cod
19	Cheesy Scrambled Eggs with Fresh Herbs	Mexican Steak Tacos	Tilapia Broccoli Platter
20	Coconut Breakfast Smoothie	Beer Pork Ribs	Parsley Scallops
21	Turkey and Green lettuce Scramble on Melba Toast	Mexican Chorizo Sausage	Blackened Chicken

CHAPTER 5:

BREAKFAST

Easy Turnip Puree

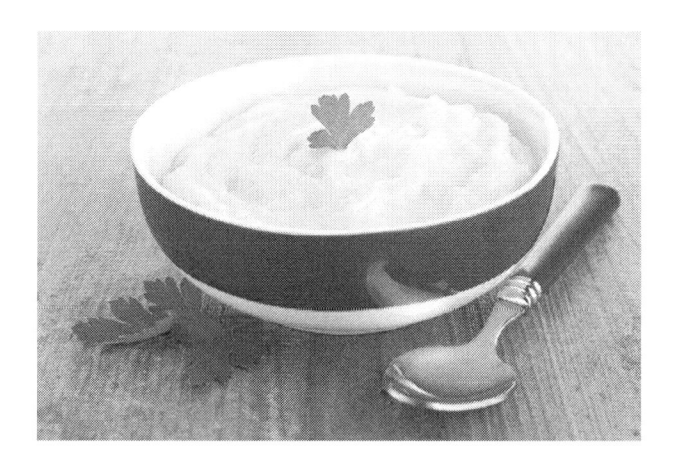

Preparation Time: 10 minutes
Cooking Time: 12 minutes
Servings: 4

Ingredients:
- 1/2 lbs. turnips, peeled and chopped
- tsp. dill
- bacon slices, cooked and chopped
- tbsp. fresh chives, chopped

Directions:
- Add turnip into the boiling water and cook for 12 minutes. Drain well and place in a food processor.
- Add dill and process until smooth.
- Transfer turnip puree into the bowl and top with bacon and chives.
- Serve and enjoy.

Nutrition:
Calories 127
Fat 6g
Carbohydrates 11.6g
Sugar 7g
Protein 6.8g
Cholesterol 16 mg

Green lettuce Bacon Breakfast Bake

Preparation Time: 10 minutes
Cooking Time: 45 minutes
Servings: 6

Ingredients:
- 10 eggs
- 3 cups baby green lettuce, chopped
- tbsp. olive oil
- 8 bacon slices, cooked and chopped
- Red bell peppers, sliced
- tbsp. chives, chopped
- Pepper
- Salt

Directions:
- Preheat the oven to 350 F.
- Spray a baking dish with cooking spray and set aside.
- Heat oil in a pan
- Add green lettuce and cook until green lettuce wilted.
- In a mixing bowl, whisk eggs and salt. Add green lettuce and chives and stir well.
- Pour egg mixture into the baking dish.
- Top with Red bell peppers and bacon and bake for 45 minutes.
- Serve and enjoy.

Nutrition:
Calories 273
Fat 20.4g
Carbohydrates 3.1g
Sugar 1.7g
Protein 19.4g
Cholesterol 301 mg

Healthy Green lettuce Tomato Muffins

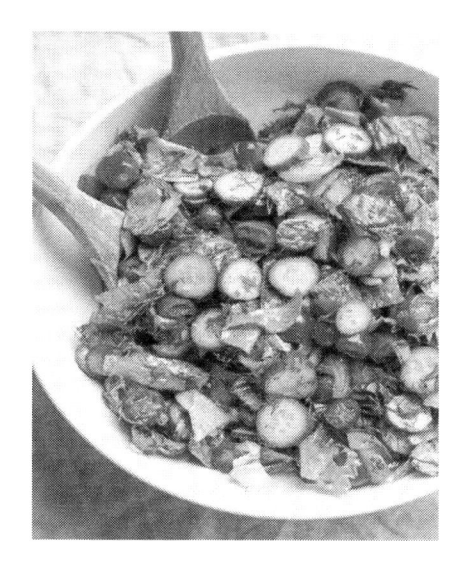

Preparation Time: 10 minutes
Cooking Time: 20 minutes
Servings: 12

Ingredients:

- 12 eggs
- 1/2 tsp. Italian seasoning
- 1 cup Red bell peppers, chopped
- 4 tbsp. water
- 1 cup fresh green lettuce, chopped
- Pepper
- Salt

Directions:

- Preheat the oven to 350 F. Spray a muffin tray with cooking spray and set aside.
- In a mixing bowl, whisk eggs with water, Italian seasoning, pepper, and salt.
- Add green lettuce and Red bell peppers and stir well.
- Pour egg mixture into the prepared muffin tray and bake for 20 minutes.
- Serve and enjoy.

Nutrition:
Calories 67
Fat 4.5g
Carbohydrates 1g
Sugar 0.8g
Protein 5.7g
Cholesterol 164 mg

Chicken Egg Breakfast Muffins

Preparation Time: 10 minutes
Cooking Time: 15 minutes
Servings: 12

Ingredients:
- 10 eggs
- 1 cup cooked chicken, chopped
- 3 tbsp. green onions, chopped
- 1/4 tsp. garlic powder
- Pepper
- Salt

Directions:
- Preheat the oven to 400 F.
- Spray a muffin tray with cooking spray and set aside.
- In a large bowl, whisk eggs with garlic powder, pepper, and salt.
- Add remaining ingredients and stir well.
- Pour egg mixture into the muffin tray and bake for 15 minutes.
- Serve and enjoy.

Nutrition:
Calories 71
Fat 4 g
Carbohydrates 0.4g
Sugar 0.3g
Protein 8g
Cholesterol 145 mg

Breakfast Egg Salad

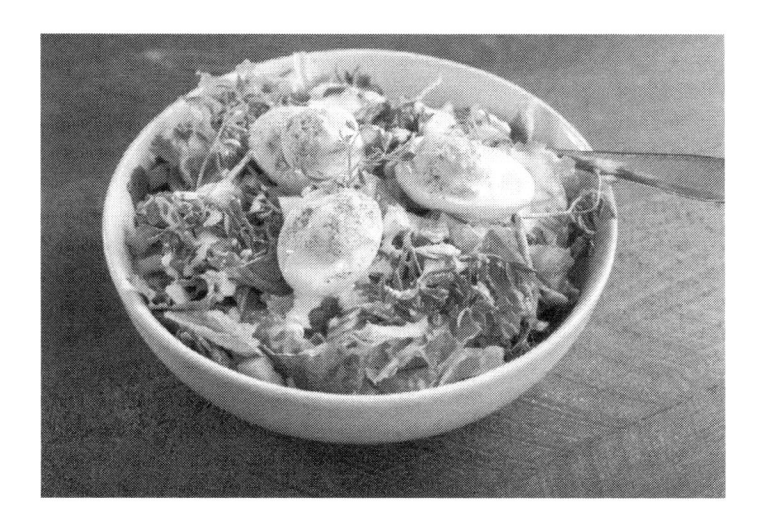

Preparation Time: 10 minutes
Cooking Time: 5 minutes
Servings: 4

Ingredients:
- 6 eggs, hard-boiled, peeled and chopped
- 1 tbsp. fresh dill, chopped
- 4 tbsp. mayonnaise
- Pepper
- Salt

Directions:
- Add all ingredients into the large bowl and stir to mix. Serve and enjoy.

Nutrition:
Calories 140
Fat 10g
Carbohydrates 4g
Sugar 1g
Protein 8g
Cholesterol 245 mg

Vegetable Tofu Scramble

Preparation Time: 10 minutes
Cooking Time: 7 minutes
Servings: 2

Ingredients:
- 1/2 block firm tofu, crumbled
- 1/4 tsp. ground cumin
- tbsp. turmeric
- cup green lettuce
- 1/4 cup zucchini, chopped
- tbsp. olive oil
- tomato, chopped
- tbsp. chives, chopped
- tbsp. coriander, chopped
- Pepper
- Salt

Directions:
- Heat oil in a pan over medium heat
- Add tomato, zucchini, and green lettuce and sauté for 2 minutes.
- Add tofu, cumin, turmeric, pepper, and salt and sauté for 5 minutes.
- Top with chives, and coriander.
- Serve and enjoy.

Nutrition:
Calories 101
Fat 8.5 g
Carbohydrates 5.1g
Sugar 1.4g
Protein 3.1g
Cholesterol 0 mg

Cheese Coconut Pancakes

Preparation Time: 10 minutes
Cooking Time: 5 minutes
Servings: 1

Ingredients:
- 2 eggs
- packet stevia
- 1/2 tsp. cinnamon
- oz. cream cheese
- tbsp. coconut flour
- 1/2 tsp. vanilla

Directions:
- Add all ingredients into the bowl and blend until smooth.
- Spray pan with cooking spray and heat over medium-high heat.
- Pour batter on the hot pan and make two pancakes.
- Cook pancake until lightly brown from both the sides.
- Serve and enjoy.

Nutrition:
Calories 386
Fat 30g
Carbohydrates 12g
Sugar 1g
Protein 16g
Cholesterol 389 mg

Cheesy Scrambled Eggs with Fresh Herbs

Preparation Time: 15 minutes
Cooking Time: 10 minutes
Servings: 4

Ingredients:
- Eggs – 3
- Egg whites – 2
- Cream cheese – 1/2 cup
- Unsweetened rice milk – 1/4 cup
- Chopped scallion – 1 Tbsp. green part only
- Chopped fresh tarragon – 1 Tbsp.
- Unsalted butter – 2 Tbsps.
- Ground black pepper to taste

Directions:
- In a bowl, whisk the eggs, egg whites, cream cheese, rice milk, scallions, and tarragon until mixed and smooth.
- Melt the butter in a skillet.
- Pour in the egg mixture and cook, stirring, for 5 minutes or until the eggs are thick and curds creamy.
- Season with pepper and serve.

Nutrition:
Calories: 221
Fat: 19g
Carb: 3g
Phosphorus: 119mg
Potassium: 140mg
Sodium: 193mg
Protein: 8g

Coconut Breakfast Smoothie

Preparation Time: 5 minutes
Cooking Time: 5 minutes
Servings: 1

Ingredients:
- 1/4 cup whey protein powder
- 1/2 cup coconut milk
- 5 drops liquid stevia
- tbsp. coconut oil
- tsp. vanilla
- tbsp. coconut butter
- 1/4 cup water
- 1/2 cup ice

Directions:
- Add all ingredients into the blender and blend until smooth.
- Serve and enjoy.

Nutrition:
Calories 560
Fat 45g
Carbohydrates 12g
Sugar 4g
Protein 25g
Cholesterol 60 mg

Turkey and Green lettuce Scramble on Melba Toast

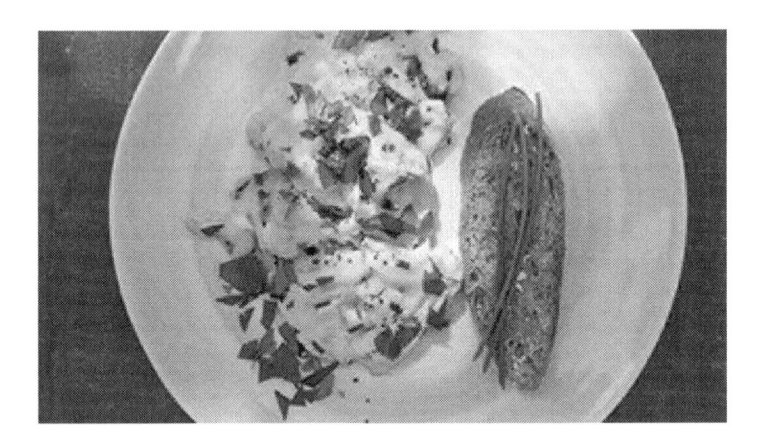

Preparation Time: 2 minutes
Cooking Time: 15 minutes
Servings: 2

Ingredients:

- Extra virgin olive oil – 1 tsp.
- Raw green lettuce – 1 cup
- Garlic – 1/2 clove, minced
- Nutmeg – 1 tsp. grated
- Cooked and diced turkey breast – 1 cup
- Melba toast – 4 slices
- Balsamic vinegar – 1 tsp.

Directions:

- Heat a skillet over medium heat and add oil.
- Add turkey and heat through for 6 to 8 minutes.
- Add green lettuce, garlic, and nutmeg and stir-fry for 6 minutes more.
- Plate up the Melba toast and top with green lettuce and turkey scramble.
- Drizzle with balsamic vinegar and serve.

Nutrition:
Calories: 301
Fat: 19g
Carb: 12g
Phosphorus: 215mg
Potassium: 269mg
Sodium: 360mg
Protein: 19g

Vegetable Omelet

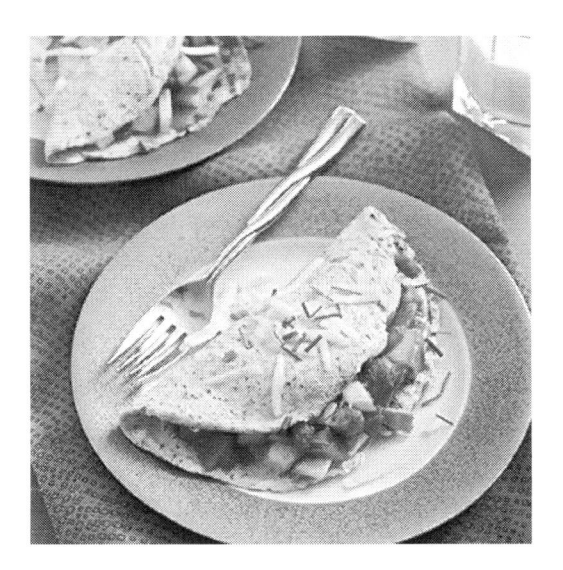

Preparation Time: 15 minutes
Cooking Time: 10 minutes
Servings: 3

Ingredients:
- Egg whites – 4
- Egg – 1
- Chopped fresh parsley – 2 Tbsps.
- Water – 2 Tbsps.
- Olive oil spray
- Chopped and boiled red bell pepper – 1/2 cup
- Chopped scallion – 1/4 cup, both green and white parts
- Ground black pepper

Directions:
- Whisk together the egg, egg whites, parsley, and water until well blended. Set aside.
- Spray a skillet with olive oil spray and place over medium heat.
- Sauté the peppers and scallion for 3 minutes or until softened.
- Pour the egg mixture into the skillet over vegetables and cook, swirling the skillet, for 2 minutes or until the edges start to set. Cook until set.
- Season with black pepper and serve.

Nutrition:
Calories: 77
Fat: 3g
Carb: 2g
Phosphorus: 67mg

Potassium: 194mg
Sodium: 229mg
Protein: 12g

Mexican Style Burritos

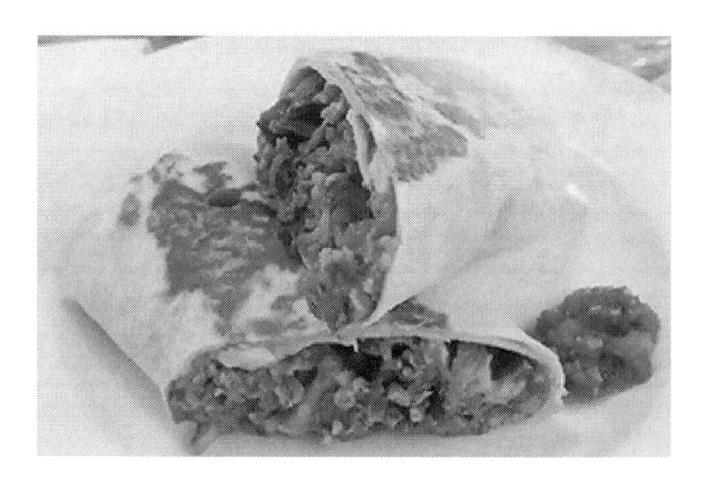

Preparation Time: 5 minutes
Cooking Time: 15 minutes
Servings: 2

Ingredients:
- Olive oil – 1 Tbsp.
- Corn tortillas – 2
- Red onion – 1/4 cup, chopped
- Red bell peppers – 1/4 cup, chopped
- Red chili – 1/2, deseeded and chopped
- Eggs – 2
- Juice of 1 lime
- Cilantro – 1 Tbsp. chopped

Directions:
- Turn the broiler to medium heat and place the tortillas underneath for 1 to 2 minutes on each side or until lightly toasted.
- Remove and keep the broiler on.
- Heat the oil in a skillet and sauté onion, chili and bell peppers for 5 to 6 minutes or until soft.
- Crack the eggs over the top of the onions and peppers and place skillet under the broiler for 5 to 6 minutes or until the eggs are cooked.
- Serve half the eggs and vegetables on top of each tortilla and sprinkle with cilantro and lime juice to serve.

Nutrition:
Calories: 202
Fat: 13g
Carb: 19g
Phosphorus: 184mg
Potassium: 233mg
Sodium: 77mg
Protein: 9g

Bulgur, Couscous and Buckwheat Cereal

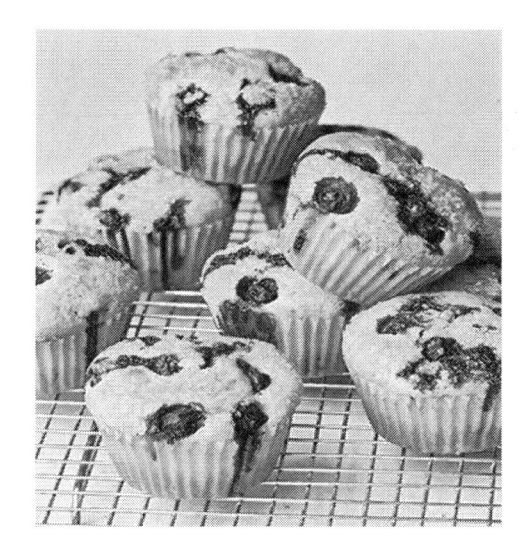

Preparation Time: 10 minutes
Cooking Time: 25 minutes
Servings: 4

Ingredients:
- Water – 2 1/4 cups
- Vanilla rice milk – 1 1/4 cups
- Uncooked bulgur – 6 Tbsps.
- Uncooked whole buckwheat – 2 Tbsps.
- Sliced apple – 1 cup
- Plain uncooked couscous – 6 Tbsps.
- Ground cinnamon – 1/2 tsp.

Directions:
- In a saucepan, heat the water and milk over medium heat.
- Bring to a boil, and add the bulgur, buckwheat, and apple.

- Reduce the heat to low and simmer, occasionally stirring until the bulgur is tender, about 20 to 25 minutes.
- Remove the saucepan from the heat and stir in the couscous and cinnamon.
- Let the saucepan stand, covered, for 10 minutes.
- Fluff the cereal with a fork before serving.

Nutrition:
Calories: 159
Fat: 1g
Carb: 34g
Phosphorus: 130mg
Potassium: 116mg
Sodium: 33mg
Protein: 4g

Sweet Pancakes

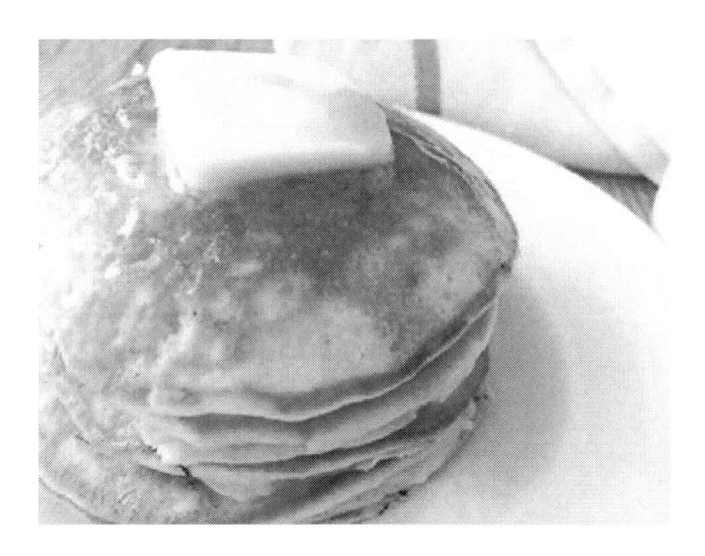

Preparation Time: 10 minutes
Cooking Time: 5 minutes
Servings: 5

Ingredients:
- All-purpose flour – 1 cup
- Granulated sugar – 1 Tbsp.
- Baking powder – 2 tsps.
- Egg whites – 2
- Almond milk - 1 cup

- Olive oil - 2 Tbsps.
- Maple extract – 1 Tbsp.

Directions:
- Mix the flour, sugar and baking powder in a bowl.
- Make a well in the center and place to one side.
- In another bowl, mix the egg whites, milk, oil, and maple extract.
- Add the egg mixture to the well and gently mix until a batter is formed.
- Heat skillet over medium heat.
- Add 1/5 of the batter to the pan and cook 2 minutes on each side or until the pancake is golden.
- Repeat with the remaining batter and serve.

Nutrition:
Calories: 178
Fat: 6g
Carb: 25g
Phosphorus: 116mg
Potassium: 126mg
Sodium: 297mg
Protein: 6g

Breakfast Smoothie

Preparation Time: 15 minutes
Cooking Time: 0 minutes
Servings: 2

Ingredients:
- Frozen blueberries – 1 cup
- Pineapple chunks – 1/2 cup
- English cucumber – 1/2 cup
- Apple – 1/2
- Water – 1/2 cup

Directions:
- Put the pineapple, blueberries, cucumber, apple, and water in a blender and blend until thick and smooth.
- Pour into 2 glasses and serve.

Nutrition:
Calories: 87
Fat: g

Carb: 22g
Phosphorus: 28mg
Potassium: 192mg
Sodium: 3mg
Protein: 0.7g

Buckwheat and Grapefruit Porridge

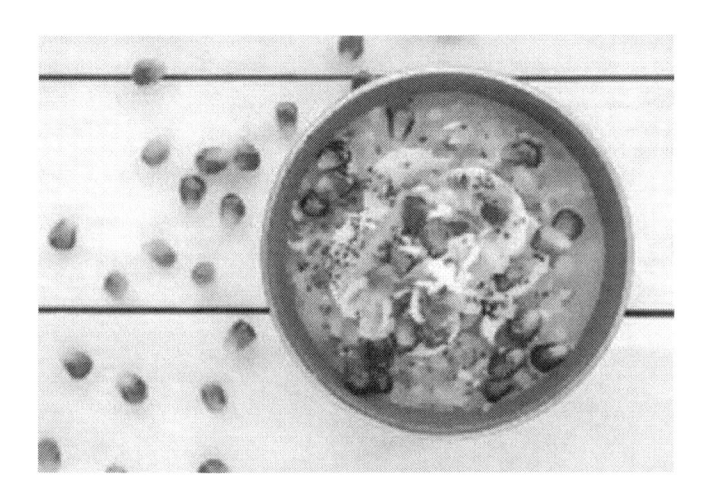

Preparation Time: 5 minutes
Cooking Time: 20 minutes
Servings: 2

Ingredients:
- Buckwheat – 1/2 cup
- Grapefruit – 1/4, chopped
- Honey – 1 Tbsp.
- Almond milk – 1 1/2 cups
- Water – 2 cups

Directions:
- Bring the water to a boil on the stove. Add the buckwheat and place the lid on the pan.
- Lower heat slightly and simmer for 7 to 10 minutes, checking to ensure water does not dry out.
- When most of the water is absorbed, remove and set aside for 5 minutes.
- Drain any excess water from the pan and stir in almond milk, heating through for 5 minutes.
- Add the honey and grapefruit.
- Serve.

Nutrition:
Calories: 231
Fat: 4g
Carb: 43g
Phosphorus: 165mg
Potassium: 370mg
Sodium: 135mg

Egg and Veggie Muffins

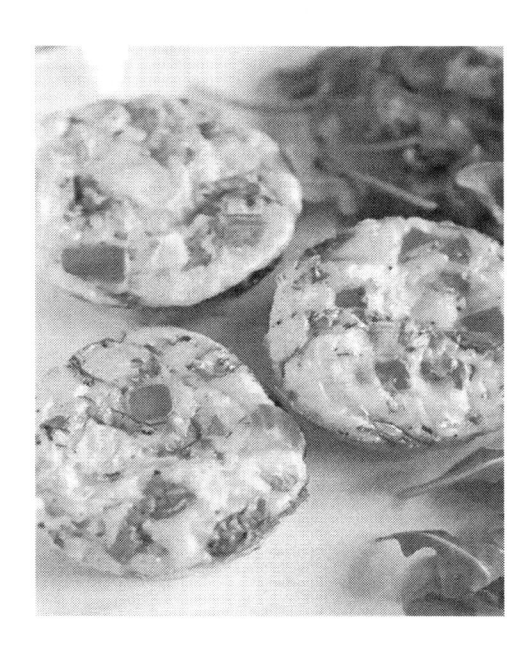

Preparation Time: 15 minutes
Cooking Time: 20 minutes
Servings: 4

Ingredients:
- Cooking spray
- Eggs – 4
- Unsweetened rice milk – 2 Tbsp.
- Sweet onion – 1/2, chopped
- Red bell pepper – 1/2, chopped
- Pinch red pepper flakes
- Pinch ground black pepper

Directions:
- Preheat the oven to 350F.
- Spray 4 muffin pans with cooking spray. Set aside.

- In a bowl, whisk together the milk, eggs, onion, red pepper, parsley, red pepper flakes, and black pepper until mixed.
- Pour the egg mixture into prepared muffin pans.
- Bake until the muffins are puffed and golden, about 18 to 20 minutes.
- serve

Nutrition:
Calories: 84
Fat: 5g
Carb: 3g
Phosphorus: 110mg
Potassium: 117mg
Sodium: 75mg
Protein: 7g

Salad with Vinaigrette

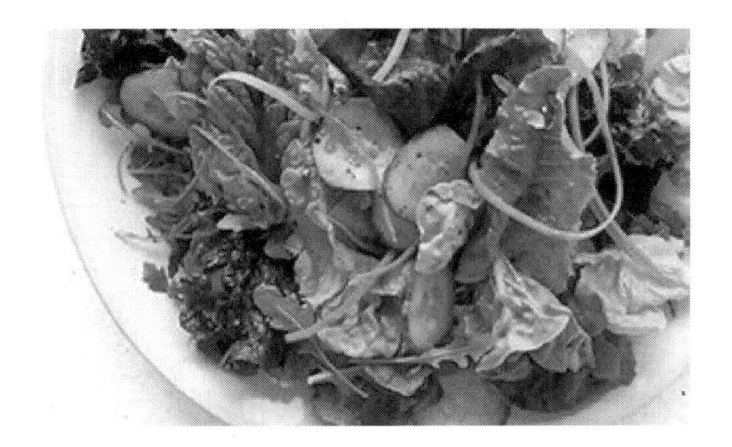

Preparation Time: 25 minutes
Cooking Time: 0 minutes
Servings: 4

Ingredients:

For the vinaigrette:
- Olive oil – 1/2 cup
- Balsamic vinegar - 4 Tbsps.
- Chopped fresh oregano – 2 Tbsps.
- Pinch red pepper flakes
- Ground black pepper

For the salad
- Shredded green leaf lettuce – 4 cups
- Carrot – 1, shredded
- Fresh green beans – ¾ cup, cut into 1-inch pieces
- Large radishes – 3, sliced thin

Directions:
- To make the vinaigrette: put the vinaigrette Ingredients in a bowl and whisk.
- To make the salad, in a bowl, toss together the carrot, lettuce, green beans, and radishes.
- Add the vinaigrette to the vegetables and toss to coat.
- Arrange the salad on plates and serve.

Nutrition:
Calories: 273
Fat: 27g
Carb: 7g
Phosphorus: 30mg
Potassium: 197mg
Sodium: 27mg
Protein: 1g

Salad with Lemon Dressing

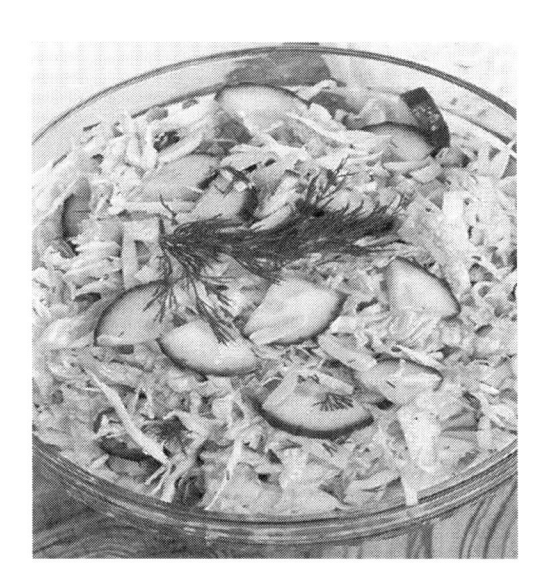

Preparation Time: 10 minutes
Cooking Time: 0 minutes
Servings: 4

Ingredients:
- Heavy cream – 1/4 cup
- Freshly squeezed lemon juice – 1/4 cup
- Granulated sugar – 2 Tbsps.
- Chopped fresh dill – 2 Tbsps.
- Finely chopped scallion – 2 Tbsps. green part only
- Ground black pepper – 1/4 tsp.
- English cucumber – 1, sliced thin
- Shredded green cabbage – 2 cups

Directions:
- In a small bowl, stir together the lemon juice, cream, sugar, dill, scallion, and pepper until well blended.
- In a large bowl, toss together the cucumber and cabbage.
- Place the salad in the refrigerator and chill for 1 hour.
- Stir before serving.

Nutrition:
Calories: 99
Fat: 6g
Carb: 13g
Phosphorus: 38mg
Potassium: 200mg
Sodium: 14mg
Protein: 2g

Shrimp with Salsa

Preparation Time: 15 minutes
Cooking Time: 10 minutes
Servings: 4

Ingredients:
- Olive oil – 2 Tbsp.
- Large shrimp – 6 ounces, peeled and deveined, tails left on
- Minced garlic – 1 tsp.
- Chopped English cucumber – 1/2 cup
- Chopped mango – 1/2 cup
- Zest of 1 lime
- Juice of 1 lime
- Ground black pepper
- Lime wedges for garnish

Directions:
- Soak 4 wooden skewers in water for 30 minutes.
- Preheat the barbecue to medium heat.
- In a bowl, toss together the olive oil, shrimp, and garlic.
- Thread the shrimp onto the skewers, about 4 shrimp per skewer.
- In a bowl, stir together the mango, cucumber, lime zest, and lime juice, and season the salsa lightly with pepper. Set aside.
- Grill the shrimp for 10 minutes, turning once or until the shrimp is opaque and cooked through.
- Season the shrimp lightly with pepper.
- Serve the shrimp on the cucumber salsa with lime wedges on the side.

Nutrition:
Calories: 120
Fat: 8g
Carb: 4g
Phosphorus: 91mg
Potassium: 129mg
Sodium: 60mg
Protein: 9g

Pesto Pork Chops

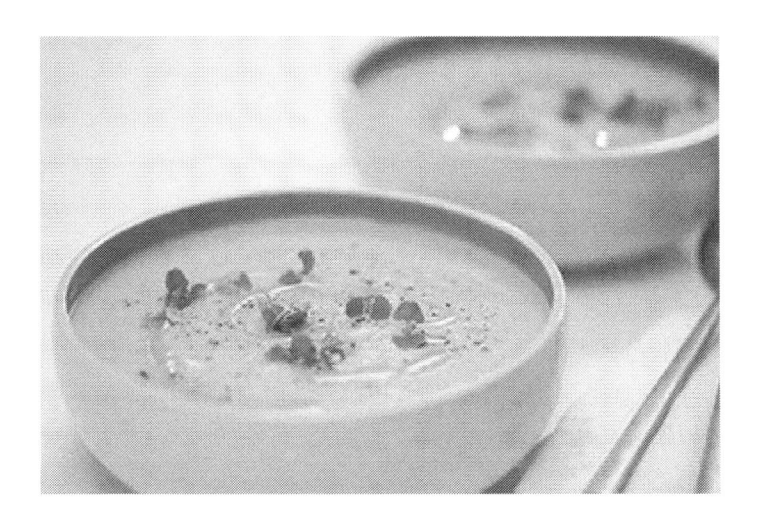

Preparation Time: 20 minutes
Cooking Time: 20 minutes
Servings: 4

Ingredients:
- Pork top-loin chops – 4 (3-ounce) boneless, fat trimmed
- Herb pesto – 8 tsps.

- Breadcrumbs – 1/2 cup
- Olive oil – 1 Tbsp.

Directions:
- Preheat the oven to 450F.
- Line a baking sheet with foil. Set aside.
- Rub 1 tsp. of pesto evenly over both sides of each pork chop.
- Lightly dredge each pork chop in the breadcrumbs.
- Heat the oil in a skillet.
- Brown the pork chops on each side for 5 minutes.
- Place the pork chops on the baking sheet.
- Bake for 10 minutes or until pork reaches 145F in the center.

Nutrition:
Calories: 210
Fat: 7g
Carb: 10g
Phosphorus: 179mg
Potassium: 220mg
Sodium: 148mg
Protein: 24g

Turkey Burgers

Preparation Time: 15 minutes
Cooking Time: 8 minutes
Servings: 5

Ingredients:
- 1 ripe pear, peeled, cored and chopped roughly
- 1-pound lean ground turkey
- 1 teaspoon fresh ginger, grated finely
- 2 minced garlic cloves
- 1 teaspoon fresh rosemary, minced
- 1 teaspoon fresh sage, minced
- Salt, to taste
- Freshly ground black pepper, to taste
- 1-2 tablespoons coconut oil

Directions:
- In a blender, add pear and pulse till smooth.
- Transfer the pear mixture in a large bowl with remaining ingredients except for oil and mix till well combined.
- Make small equal sized 10 patties from the mixture.
- In a heavy-bottomed frying pan, heat oil on medium heat.
- Add the patties and cook for around 4-5 minutes.
- Flip the inside and cook for approximately 2-3 minutes.

Nutrition:
Calories: 477
Fat: 15g
Carbohydrates: 26g
Fiber: 11g
Protein: 35g

CHAPTER 6:
LUNCH

Dolmas Wrap

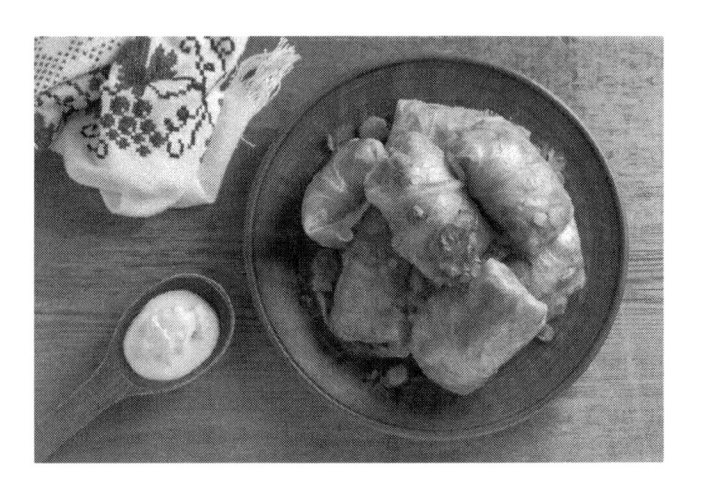

Preparation Time: 10 minutes
Cooking Time: 5 minutes
Servings: 2

Ingredients:
- 2 whole wheat wraps
- 6 dolmas (stuffed grape leaves)
- tomato, chopped
- cucumber, chopped
- oz. Greek yogurt
- ½ teaspoon minced garlic
- ¼ cup lettuce, chopped
- oz. Feta, crumbled

Directions:
- In the mixing bowl combine together chopped tomato, cucumber, Greek yogurt, minced garlic, lettuce, and Feta.
- When the mixture is homogenous transfer it in the center of every wheat wrap.
- Arrange dolma over the vegetable mixture.
- Carefully wrap the wheat wraps.

Nutrition:
calories 341, fat 12.9, fiber 9.2, carbs 52.4, protein 13.2 Phosphorus: 110mg Potassium: 117mg Sodium: 75mg

Salad al Tonno

Preparation Time: 15 minutes
Cooking Time: 0 minutes
Servings: 2

Ingredients:
- ½ cup lettuce leaves, teared
- ½ cup cherry Red bell peppers, halved
- ½ teaspoon garlic powder
- ½ teaspoon salt
- ½ teaspoon ground black pepper
- tablespoon lemon juice
- 6 oz. tuna, canned, drained

Directions:
- Chop the tuna roughly and put it in the salad bowl.
- Add cherry Red bell peppers, lettuce leaves, salt, garlic powder, ground black pepper. Lemon juice, and olive oil.
- Give a good shake to the salad.
- Salad can be stored in the fridge for up to 3 hours.

Nutrition: calories 235, fat 12, fiber 1, carbs 6.5, protein 23.4 Phosphorus: 120mg Potassium: 217mg Sodium: 75mg

Arlecchino Rice Salad

Preparation Time: 10 minutes
Cooking Time: 15 minutes
Servings: 3

Ingredients:
- ½ cup white rice, dried
- cup chicken stock
- zucchini, shredded
- tablespoons capers
- carrot, shredded
- tomato, chopped
- tablespoon apple cider vinegar
- ½ teaspoon salt

- tablespoons fresh parsley, chopped
- tablespoon canola oil

Directions:
- Put rice in the pan.
- Add chicken stock and boil it with the closed lid for 15-20 minutes or until rice absorbs all water.
- Meanwhile, in the mixing bowl combine together shredded zucchini, capers, carrot, and tomato.
- Add fresh parsley.
- Make the dressing: mix up together canola oil, salt, and apple cider vinegar.
- Chill the cooked rice little and add it in the salad bowl to the vegetables.
- Add dressing and mix up salad well.

Nutrition:
calories 183,
fat 5.3,
fiber 2.1,
carbs 30.4,
protein 3.8
Phosphorus: 110mg
Potassium: 117mg
Sodium: 75mg

Sauteed Chickpea and Lentil Mix

Preparation Time: 10 minutes
Cooking Time: 50 minutes
Servings: 4

Ingredients:
- cup chickpeas, half-cooked
- cup lentils
- 5 cups chicken stock
- ½ cup fresh cilantro, chopped
- teaspoon salt
- ½ teaspoon chili flakes
- ¼ cup onion, diced
- tablespoon tomato paste

Directions:
- Place chickpeas in the pan.
- Add water, salt, and chili flakes.
- Boil the chickpeas for 30 minutes over the medium heat.

- Then add diced onion, lentils, and tomato paste. Stir well.
- Close the lid and cook the mix for 15 minutes.
- After this, add chopped cilantro, stir the meal well and cook it for 5 minutes more.
- Let the cooked lunch chill little before serving.

Nutrition: calories 370, fat 4.3, fiber 23.7, carbs 61.6, protein 23.2 Phosphorus: 110mg Potassium: 117mg Sodium: 75mg

Crazy Japanese Potato and Beef Croquettes

Preparation Time: 10 minutes
Cooking Time: 20 minutes
Servings: 10

Ingredients:
- 3 medium russet potatoes, peeled and chopped
- tablespoon almond butter
- tablespoon vegetable oil
- onions, diced
- ¾ pound ground beef
- teaspoons light coconut aminos
- All-purpose flour for coating
- eggs, beaten
- Panko bread crumbs for coating
- ½ cup oil, frying

Directions:
- Take a saucepan and place it over medium-high heat; add potatoes and sunflower seeds water, boil for 16 minutes.
- Remove water and put potatoes in another bowl, add almond butter and mash the potatoes.
- Take a frying pan and place it over medium heat, add 1 tablespoon oil and let it heat up.
- Add onions and stir fry until tender.
- Add coconut aminos to beef to onions.
- Keep frying until beef is browned.
- Mix the beef with the potatoes evenly.
- Take another frying pan and place it over medium heat; add half a cup of oil.
- Form croquettes using the mashed potato mixture and coat them with flour, then eggs and finally breadcrumbs.
- Fry patties until golden on all sides.
- Enjoy!

Nutrition: Calories: 239 Fat: 4g Carbohydrates: 20g Protein: 10g Phosphorus: 120mg Potassium: 107mg Sodium: 75mg

Traditional Black Bean Chili

Preparation Time: 10 minutes
Cooking Time: 4 hours
Servings: 4

Ingredients:
- ½ cups red bell pepper, chopped
- cup yellow onion, chopped
- ½ cups mushrooms, sliced
- tablespoon olive oil
- tablespoon chili powder
- garlic cloves, minced
- teaspoon chipotle chili pepper, chopped
- ½ teaspoon cumin, ground
- 16 ounces canned black beans, drained and rinsed
- tablespoons cilantro, chopped
- cup Red bell peppers, chopped

Directions:
- Add red bell peppers, onion, dill, mushrooms, chili powder, garlic, chili pepper, cumin, black beans, and Red bell peppers to your Slow Cooker.
- Stir well.
- Place lid and cook on HIGH for 4 hours.
- Sprinkle cilantro on top.
- Serve and enjoy!

Nutrition: Calories: 211 Fat: 3g Carbohydrates: 22g Protein: 5g Phosphorus: 90mg Potassium: 107mg Sodium: 75mg

Green Palak Paneer

Preparation Time: 5 minutes
Cooking Time: 10 minutes
Servings: 4

Ingredients:
- 1-pound green lettuce
- 2 cups cubed paneer (vegan)
- 2 tablespoons coconut oil
- teaspoon cumin
- chopped up onion
- 1-2 teaspoons hot green chili minced up
- teaspoon minced garlic
- 15 cashews
- 4 tablespoons almond milk
- teaspoon Garam masala
- Flavored vinegar as needed

Directions:
- Add cashews and milk to a blender and blend well.
- Set your pot to Sauté mode and add coconut oil; allow the oil to heat up.
- Add cumin seeds, garlic, green chilies, ginger and sauté for 1 minute.
- Add onion and sauté for 2 minutes.
- Add chopped green lettuce, flavored vinegar and a cup of water.
- Lock up the lid and cook on HIGH pressure for 10 minutes.
- Quick-release the pressure.
- Add ½ cup of water and blend to a paste.
- Add cashew paste, paneer and Garam Masala and stir thoroughly.
- Serve over hot rice!

Nutrition:
Calories: 367
Fat: 26g
Carbohydrates: 21g
Protein: 16g
Phosphorus: 110mg
Potassium: 117mg
Sodium: 75mg

Cucumber Sandwich

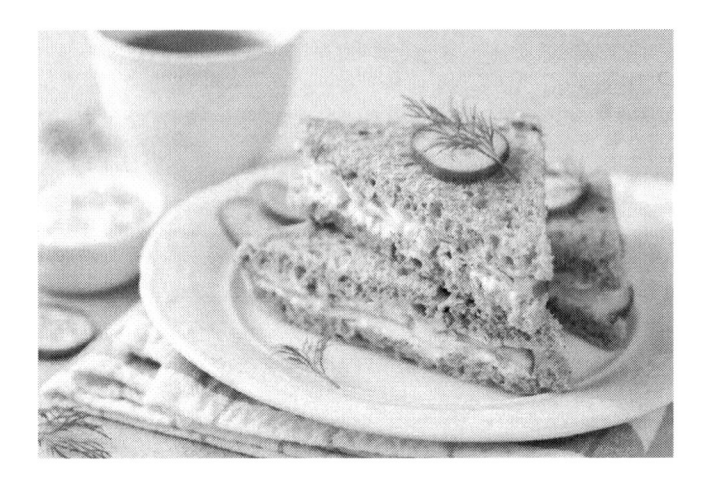

Preparation Time: 1 hour
Cooking Time: 5 minutes
Servings: 2

Ingredients:
- 6 tsp. of cream cheese
- 1 pinch of dried dill weed
- 3 tsp. of mayonnaise
- .25 tsp. dry Italian dressing mix
- 4 slices of white bread
- .5 of a cucumber

Directions:
- Prepare the cucumber and cut it into slices.
- Mix cream cheese, mayonnaise, and Italian dressing. Chill for one hour.
- Distribute the mixture onto the white bread slices.
- Place cucumber slices on top and sprinkle with the dill weed.
- Cut in halves and serve.

Nutrition:
Calories: 143
Fat: 6g
Carbs: 16.7g
Protein: 4g
Sodium: 255mg
Potassium: 127mg
Phosphorus: 64mg

Pizza Pitas

Preparation Time: 10 minutes
Cooking Time: 10 minutes
Servings: 1

Ingredients:
- .33 cup of mozzarella cheese
- 2 pieces of pita bread, 6 inches in size
- 6 tsp. of chunky tomato sauce
- 2 cloves of garlic (minced)
- .25 cups of onion, chopped small
- .25 tsp. of red pepper flakes
- .25 cup of bell pepper, chopped small
- 2 ounces of ground pork, lean
- No-stick oil spray
- .5 tsp. of fennel seeds

Directions:
- Preheat oven to 400.
- Put the garlic, ground meat, pepper flakes, onion, and bell pepper in a pan. Sauté until cooked.
- Grease a flat baking pan and put pitas on it. Use the mixture to spread on the pita bread.
- Spread one tablespoon of the tomato sauce and top with cheese.
- Bake for five to eight minutes, until the cheese is bubbling.

Nutrition:
Calories: 284
Fat: 10g
Carbs: 34g
Protein: 16g
Sodium: 795mg
Potassium: 706mg
Phosphorus: 416mg

Lettuce Wraps with Chicken

Preparation Time: 10 minutes
Cooking Time: 15 minutes
Servings: 4

Ingredients:
- 8 lettuce leaves
- .25 cups of fresh cilantro
- .25 cups of mushroom
- 1 tsp. of five spices seasoning
- .25 cups of onion
- 6 tsp. of rice vinegar
- 2 tsp. of hoisin
- 6 tsp. of oil (canola)
- 3 tsp. of oil (sesame)
- 2 tsp. of garlic
- 2 scallions
- 8 ounces of cooked chicken breast

Directions:
- Mince together the cooked chicken and the garlic. Chop up the onions, cilantro, mushrooms, and scallions.
- Use a skillet overheat, combine chicken to all remaining ingredients, minus the lettuce leaves. Cook for fifteen minutes, stirring occasionally.
- Place .25 cups of the mixture into each leaf of lettuce.
- Wrap the lettuce around like a burrito and eat.

Nutrition:
Calories: 84
Fat: 4g
Carbs: 9g
Protein: 5.9g
Sodium: 618mg
Potassium: 258mg
Phosphorus: 64mg

Turkey Pinwheels

Preparation Time: 10 minutes
Cooking Time: 15 minutes
Servings: 6

Ingredients:
- 6 toothpicks
- 8 oz. of spring mix salad greens
- 1 ten-inch tortilla
- 2 ounces of thinly sliced deli turkey
- 9 tsp. of whipped cream cheese
- 1 roasted red bell pepper

Directions:
- Cut the red bell pepper into ten strips about a quarter-inch thick.
- Spread the whipped cream cheese on the tortilla evenly.
- Add the salad greens to create a base layer and then lay the turkey on top of it.
- Space out the red bell pepper strips on top of the turkey.
- Tuck the end and begin rolling the tortilla inward.
- Use the toothpicks to hold the roll into place and cut it into six pieces.
- Serve with the swirl facing upward.

Nutrition:
Calories: 206
Fat: 9g
Carbs: 21g
Protein: 9g
Sodium: 533mg
Potassium: 145mg
Phosphorus: 47mg

Chicken Tacos

Preparation Time: 5 minutes
Cooking Time: 20 minutes
Servings: 4

Ingredients:
- 8 corn tortillas
- 1.5 tsp. of Sodium-free taco seasoning
- 1 juiced lime
- .5 cups of cilantro
- 2 green onions, chopped
- 8 oz. of iceberg or romaine lettuce, shredded or chopped
- .25 cup of sour cream
- 1 pound of boneless and skinless chicken breast

Directions:
- Cook chicken, by boiling, for twenty minutes. Shred or chop cooked chicken into fine bite-sized pieces.
- Mix the seasoning and lime juice with the chicken.
- Put chicken mixture and lettuce in tortillas.
- Top with the green onions, cilantro, and sour cream.

Nutrition:
Calories: 260
Fat: 3g
Carbs: 36g
Protein: 23g
Sodium: 922mg
Potassium: 445mg
Phosphorus: 357mg

Tuna Twist

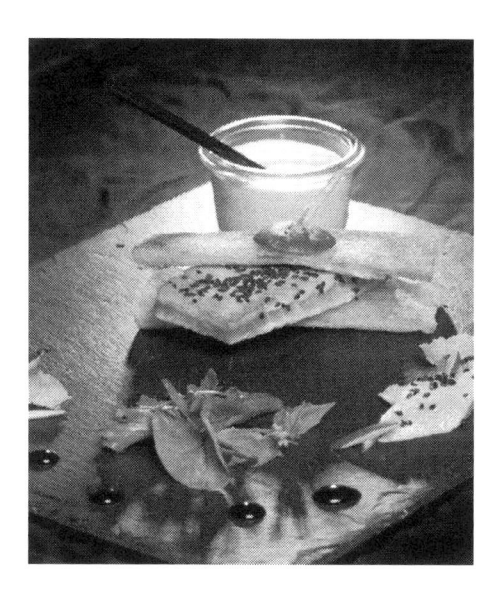

Preparation Time: 10 minutes
Cooking Time: 30 minutes
Servings: 4

Ingredients:
- 1 can of unsalted or water packaged tuna, drained
- 6 tsp. of vinegar
- .5 cup of cooked peas
- .5 cup celery (chopped)
- 3 tsp. of dried dill weed
- 12 oz. cooked macaroni
- .75 cup of mayonnaise

Directions:
- Stir together the macaroni, vinegar, and mayonnaise together until blended and smooth.
- Stir in remaining ingredients.
- Chill before serving.

Nutrition:
Calories: 290
Fat: 10g
Carbs: 32g
Protein: 16g
Sodium: 307mg
Potassium: 175mg
Phosphorus: 111mg

Ciabatta Rolls with Chicken Pesto

Preparation Time: 10 minutes
Cooking Time: 20 minutes
Servings: 2

Ingredients:
- 6 tsp. of Greek yogurt
- 6 tsp. of pesto
- 2 small ciabatta rolls
- 8 oz. of a shredded iceberg or romaine lettuce
- 8 oz. of cooked boneless and skinless chicken breast, shredded
- .125 tsp. of pepper

Directions:
- Combine the shredded chicken, pesto, pepper, and Greek yogurt in a medium-sized bowl.
- Slice and toast the ciabatta rolls.
- Divide the shredded chicken and pesto mixture in half and make sandwiches with the ciabatta rolls.
- Top with shredded lettuce if desired.

Nutrition:
Calories: 374
Fat: 10g
Carbs: 40g
Protein: 30g
Sodium: 522mg
Potassium: 360mg
Phosphorus: 84mg

Marinated Shrimp Pasta Salad

Preparation Time: 15 minutes
Cooking Time: 5 hours
Servings: 1

Ingredients:
- 1/4 cup of honey
- 1/4 cup of balsamic vinegar
- 1/2 of an English cucumber, cubed
- 1/2 pound of fully cooked shrimp
- 15 baby carrots

- 1.5 cups of dime-sized cut cauliflower
- 4 stalks of celery, diced
- 1/2 large yellow bell pepper (diced)
- 1/2 red onion (diced)
- 1/2 large red bell pepper (diced)
- 12 ounces of uncooked tri-color pasta (cooked)
- 3/4 cup of olive oil
- 3 tsp. of mustard (Dijon)
- 1/2 tsp. of garlic (powder)
- 1/2 tsp. pepper

Directions:
- Cut vegetables and put them in a bowl with the shrimp.
- Whisk together the honey, balsamic vinegar, garlic powder, pepper, and Dijon mustard in a small bowl. While still whisking, slowly add the oil and whisk it all together.
- Add the cooked pasta to the bowl with the shrimp and vegetables and mix it.
- Toss the sauce to coat the pasta, shrimp, and vegetables evenly.
- Cover and chill for a minimum of five hours before serving. Stir and serve while chilled.

Nutrition:
Calories: 205
Fat: 13g
Carbs: 10g
Protein: 12g
Sodium: 363mg
Potassium: 156mg
Phosphorus: 109mg

Peanut Butter and Jelly Grilled Sandwich

Preparation Time: 5 minutes
Cooking Time: 5 minutes
Servings: 1

Ingredients:
- 2 tsp. butter (unsalted)
- 6 tsp. butter (peanut)
- 3 tsp. of flavored jelly
- 2 pieces of bread

Directions:
- Put the peanut butter evenly on one bread. Add the layer of jelly.
- Butter the outside of the pieces of bread.
- Add the sandwich to a frying pan and toast both sides.

Nutrition:
Calories: 300
Fat: 7g
Carbs: 49g
Protein: 8g
Sodium: 460mg
Potassium: 222mg
Phosphorus: 80mg

Grilled Onion and Pepper Jack Grilled Cheese Sandwich

Preparation Time: 5 minutes
Cooking Time: 5 minutes
Servings: 2

Ingredients:
- 1 tsp. of oil (olive)
- 6 tsp. of whipped cream cheese
- 1/2 of a medium onion
- 2 ounces of pepper jack cheese
- 4 slices of rye bread
- 2 tsp. of unsalted butter

Directions:
- Set out the butter so that it becomes soft. Slice up the onion into thin slices.
- Sauté onion slices. Continue to stir until cooked. Remove and put it to the side.
- Spread one tablespoon of the whipped cream cheese on two of the slices of bread.
- Then add grilled onions and cheese to each slice. Then top using the other two bread slices.
- Spread the softened butter on the outside of the slices of bread.
- Use the skillet to toast the sandwiches until lightly brown and the cheese is melted.

Nutrition:
Calories: 350
Fat: 18g

Carbs: 34g
Protein: 13g
Sodium: 589mg
Potassium: 184mg
Phosphorus: 226mg

Crispy Lemon Chicken

Preparation Time: 10 minutes
Cooking Time: 10 minutes
Servings: 6

Ingredients:
- 1 lb. boneless and skinless chicken breast
- ½ cup of all-purpose flour
- 1 large egg
- ½ cup of lemon juice
- 2 tbsp. of water
- ¼ tsp salt
- ¼ tsp lemon pepper
- 1 tsp of mixed herb seasoning
- 2 tbsp. of olive oil
- A few lemon slices for garnishing
- 1 tbsp. of chopped parsley (for garnishing)
- 2 cups of cooked plain white rice

Directions:
- Slice the chicken breast into thin and season with the herb, salt, and pepper.
- In a small bowl, whisk together the egg with the water.
- Keep the flour in a separate bowl.
- Dip the chicken slices in the egg bath and then into the flour.
- Heat your oil in a medium frying pan.
- Shallow fry the chicken in the pan until golden brown.
- Add the lemon juice and cook for another couple of minutes.
- Taken the chicken out of the pan and transfer on a wide dish with absorbing paper to absorb any excess oil.
- Garnish with some chopped parsley and lemon wedges on top.
- Serve with rice.

Nutrition:
Calories: 232
Carbohydrate: 24g
Protein: 18g
Fat: 8g
Sodium: 100g
Potassium: 234mg
Phosphorus: 217mg

Mexican Steak Tacos

Preparation Time: 10 minutes
Cooking Time: 15 minutes
Servings: 8

Ingredients:
- 1 pound of flank or skirt steak
- ¼ cup of fresh cilantro, chopped
- ¼ cup white onion, chopped
- 3 limes, juiced
- 3 cloves of garlic, minced
- 2 tsp of garlic powder
- 2 tbsp. of olive oil
- ½ cup of Mexican or mozzarella cheese, grated
- 1 tsp of Mexican seasoning
- 8 medium-sized (6") corn flour tortillas

Directions:
- Combine the juice from two limes, Mexican seasoning, and garlic powder in a dish or bowl and marinate the steak with it for at least half an hour in the fridge.
- In a separate bowl, combine the chopped cilantro, garlic, onion, and juice from one lime to make your salsa. Cover and keep in the fridge.
- Slice steak into thin strips and cook for approximately 3 minutes on each side.
- Preheat your oven to 350F/180C.
- Distribute evenly the steak strips in each tortilla. Top with a tablespoon of the grated cheese on top.
- Wrap each taco in aluminum foil and bake in the oven for 7-8 minutes or until cheese is melted.
- Serve warm with your cilantro salsa.

Nutrition:
Calories: 230
Carbohydrate: 19.5 g

Protein: 15 g
Fat: 11 g
Sodium: 486.75 g
Potassium: 240 mg
Phosphorus: 268 mg

Beer Pork Ribs

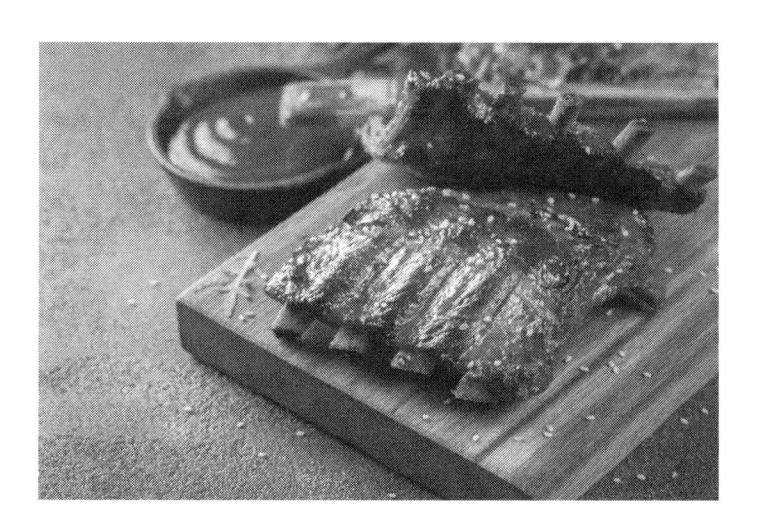

Preparation Time: 10 minutes
Cooking Time: 8 hours
Servings: 1

Ingredients:
- 2 pounds of pork ribs, cut into two units/racks
- 18 oz. of root beer
- 2 cloves of garlic, minced
- 2 tbsp. of onion powder
- 2 tbsp. of vegetable oil (optional)

Directions:
- Wrap the pork ribs with vegetable oil and place one unit on the bottom of your slow cooker with half of the minced garlic and the onion powder.
- Place the other rack on top with the rest of the garlic and onion powder.
- Pour over the root beer and cover the lid.
- Let simmer for 8 hours on low heat.
- Take off and finish optionally in a grilling pan for a nice sear.

Nutrition:
Calories: 301

Carbohydrate: 36 g
Protein: 21 g
Fat: 18 g
Sodium: 729 mg
Potassium: 200 mg
Phosphorus: 209 mg

Mexican Chorizo Sausage

Preparation Time: 10 minutes
Cooking Time: 15 minutes
Servings: 1

Ingredients:
- 2 pounds of boneless pork but coarsely ground
- 3 tbsp. of red wine vinegar
- 2 tbsp. of smoked paprika
- ½ tsp of cinnamon
- ½ tsp of ground cloves
- ¼ tsp of coriander seeds
- ¼ tsp ground ginger
- 1 tsp of ground cumin
- 3 tbsp. of brandy

Directions:
- In a large mixing bowl, combine the ground pork with the seasonings, brandy, and vinegar and mix with your hands well.
- Place the mixture into a large Ziploc bag and leave in the fridge overnight.
- Form into 15-16 patties of equal size.
- Heat the oil in a large pan and fry the patties for 5-7 minutes on each side, or until the meat inside is no longer pink and there is a light brown crust on top.
- Serve hot.

Nutrition:
Calories: 134
Carbohydrate: 0 g
Protein: 10 g
Fat: 7 g
Sodium: 40 mg
Potassium: 138 mg
Phosphorus: 128 mg

Eggplant Casserole

Preparation Time: 10 minutes
Cooking Time: 25 – 30 minutes
Servings: 4

Ingredients:
- 3 cups of eggplant, peeled and cut into large chunks
- 2 egg whites
- 1 large egg, whole
- ½ cup of unsweetened vegetable
- ¼ tsp of sage
- ½ cup of breadcrumbs
- 1 tbsp. of margarine, melted
- 1/4 tsp garlic salt

Directions:
- Preheat the oven at 350F/180C.
- Place the eggplants chunks in a medium pan, cover with a bit of water and cook with the lid covered until tender. Drain from the water and mash with a tool or fork.
- Beat the eggs with the non-dairy vegetable cream, sage, salt, and pepper. Whisk in the eggplant mush.
- Combine the melted margarine with the breadcrumbs.
- Bake in the oven for 20-25 minutes or until the casserole has a golden-brown crust.

Nutrition:
Calories: 186
Carbohydrate: 19 g
Protein: 7 g
Fat: 9 g
Sodium: 503 mg
Potassium: 230 mg
Phosphorus: 62 mg

Pizza with Chicken and Pesto

Preparation Time: 10 minutes
Cooking Time: 25 minutes
Servings: 4

Ingredients:
- 1 ready-made frozen pizza dough
- 2/3 cup cooked chicken, chopped
- 1/2 cup of orange bell pepper, diced
- 1/2 cup of green bell pepper, diced
- 1/4 cup of purple onion, chopped
- 2 tbsp. of green basil pesto
- 1 tbsp. of chives, chopped
- 1/3 cup of parmesan or Romano cheese, grated
- 1/4 cup of mozzarella cheese
- 1 tbsp. of olive oil

Directions:
- Thaw the pizza dough according to instructions on the package.
- Heat the olive oil in a pan and sauté the peppers and onions for a couple of minutes. Set aside
- Once the pizza dough has thawed, spread the Bali pesto over its surface.
- Top with half of the cheese, the peppers, the onions, and the chicken. Finish with the rest of the cheese.
- Bake at 350F/180C for approx. 20 minutes (or until crust and cheese are baked).
- Slice in triangles with a pizza cutter or sharp knife and serve.

Nutrition:
Calories: 225
Carbohydrate: 13.9 g
Protein: 11.1 g
Fat: 12 g
Sodium: 321 mg
Potassium: 174 mg
Phosphorus: 172 mg

Shrimp Quesadilla

Preparation Time: 10 minutes
Cooking Time: 10 minutes
Servings: 2

Ingredients:
- 5 oz. of shrimp, shelled and deveined
- 4 tbsp. of Mexican salsa
- 2 tbsp. of fresh cilantro, chopped
- 1 tbsp. of lemon juice
- 1 tsp of ground cumin
- 1 tsp of cayenne pepper
- 2 tbsp. of unsweetened soy yogurt or creamy tofu
- 2 medium corn flour tortillas
- 2 tbsp. of low-fat cheddar cheese

Directions:
- Mix the cilantro, cumin, lemon juice, and cayenne in a Ziploc bag to make your marinade.
- Put the shrimps and marinate for 10 minutes.
- Heat a pan over medium heat with some olive oil and toss in the shrimp with the marinade. Let cook for a couple of minutes or as soon as shrimps have turned pink and opaque.
- Add the soy cream or soft tofu to the pan and mix well. Remove from the heat and keep the marinade aside.
- Heat tortillas in the grill or microwave for a few seconds.
- Place 2 tbsp. of salsa on each tortilla. Top one tortilla with the shrimp mixture and add the cheese on top.
- Stack one tortilla against each other (with the spread salsa layer facing the shrimp mixture).
- Transfer this on a baking tray and cook for 7-8 minutes at 350F/180C to melt the cheese and crisp up the tortillas.
- Serve warm.

Nutrition:
Calories: 255
Carbohydrate: 21 g
Fat: 9 g
Protein: 24 g
Sodium: 562 g
Potassium: 235 mg
Phosphorus: 189 mg

Grilled Corn on the Cob

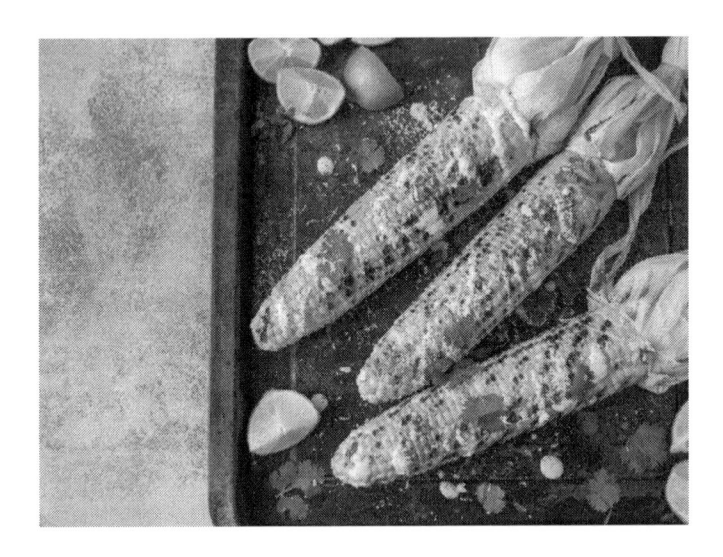

Preparation Time: 5 minutes
Cooking Time: 20 minutes
Servings: 4

Ingredients:
- 4 frozen corn on the cob, cut in half
- ½ tsp of thyme
- 1 tbsp. of grated parmesan cheese
- ¼ tsp of black pepper

Directions:
- Combine the oil, cheese, thyme, and black pepper in a bowl.
- Place the corn in the cheese/oil mix and roll to coat evenly.
- Fold all 4 pieces in aluminum foil, leaving a small open surface on top.
- Place the wrapped corns over the grill and let cook for 20 minutes.
- Serve hot.

Nutrition:
Calories: 125
Carbohydrate: 29.5 g
Protein: 2 g
Fat: 1.3 g
Sodium: 26 g
Potassium: 145 mg
Phosphorus: 91.5 mg

Couscous with Veggies

Preparation Time: 10 minutes
Cooking Time: 10 minutes
Servings: 5

Ingredients:
- ½ cup of uncooked couscous
- ¼ cup of white mushrooms, sliced
- ½ cup of red onion, chopped
- 1 garlic clove, minced
- ½ cup of frozen peas
- 2 tbsp. of dry white wine
- ½ tsp of basil
- 2 tbsp. of fresh parsley, chopped
- 1 cup water or vegetable stock
- 1 tbsp. of margarine or vegetable oil

Directions:
- Thaw the peas by setting them aside at room temperature for 15-20 minutes.
- In a medium pan, heat the margarine or vegetable oil.
- Add the onions, peas, mushroom, and garlic and sauté for around 5 minutes. Add the wine and let it evaporate.
- Add all the herbs and spices and toss well. Take off the heat and keep aside.
- In a small pot, cook the couscous with 1 cup of hot water or vegetable stock. Bring to a boil, take off the heat, and sit for a few minutes with a lid covered.
- Add the sauté veggies to the couscous and toss well.
- Serve in a serving bowl warm or cold.

Nutrition:
Calories: 110.4
Carbohydrate: 18 g
Protein: 3 g
Fat: 2 g
Sodium: 112.2 mg
Potassium: 69.6 mg
Phosphorus: 46.8 mg

Easy Egg Salad

Preparation Time: 5 minutes
Cooking Time: 8 minutes
Servings: 4

Ingredients:
- 4 large eggs
- ½ cup of sweet onion, chopped
- ¼ cup of celery, chopped
- 1 tbsp. of yellow mustard
- 1 tsp of smoked paprika
- 3 tbsp. of mayo

Directions:
- Hard boil the eggs in a small pot filled with water for approx. 7-8 minutes. Leave the eggs in the water for an extra couple of minutes before peeling.
- Peel the eggs and chop finely with a knife or tool.
- Combine all the chopped veggies with the mayo and mustard. Add in the eggs and mix well.
- Sprinkle with some smoked paprika on top.
- Serve cold with pitta, white bread slices, or lettuce wraps.

Nutrition:
Calories: 127
Carbohydrate: 6 g
Protein: 7 g
Fat: 13 g
Sodium: 170.7 mg
Potassium: 87.5 mg
Phosphorus: 101 mg

Cauliflower Rice and Coconut

Preparation Time: 20 minutes
Cooking Time: 20 minutes
Serving: 4

Ingredients:
- 3 cups cauliflower, riced
- 2/3 cups full-fat coconut milk

- 1-2 teaspoons sriracha paste
- ¼- ½ teaspoon onion powder
- Salt as needed
- Fresh basil for garnish

Directions:
- Take a pan and place it over medium-low heat
- Add all of the ingredients and stir them until fully combined
- Cook for about 5-10 minutes, making sure that the lid is on
- Remove the lid and keep cooking until there's no excess liquid
- Once the rice is soft and creamy, enjoy it!

Nutrition:
Calories: 95
Fat: 7g
Carbohydrates: 4g
Protein: 1g

Kale and Garlic Platter

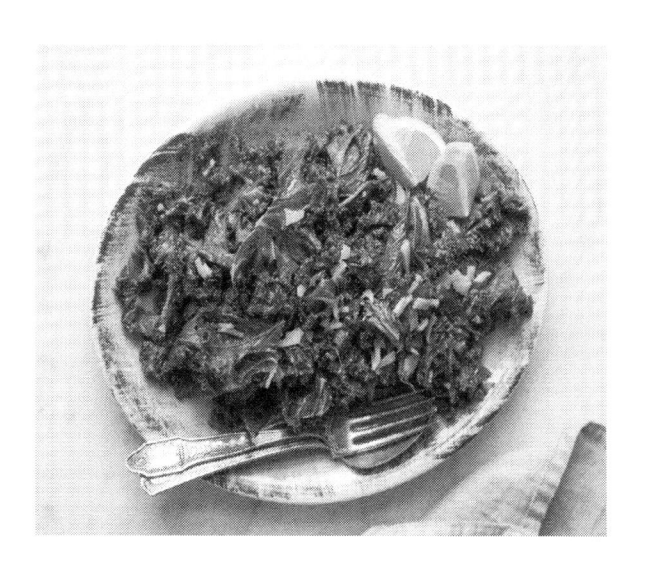

Preparation Time: 5 minutes
Cooking Time: 10 minutes
Serving: 4

Ingredients:
- bunch kale
- tablespoons olive oil
- garlic cloves, minced

Directions:
- Carefully tear the kale into bite-sized portions, making sure to remove the stem
- Discard the stems
- Place on a pot over medium heat.
- Add olive oil, let heat.
- Add garlic and stir for 2 minutes
- Add kale and cook for 5-10 minutes
- Serve!

Nutrition:
Calories: 121
Fat: 8g
Carbohydrates: 5g
Protein: 4g

Blistered Beans and Almond

Preparation Time: 10 minutes
Cooking Time: 20 minutes
Serving: 4

Ingredients:
- 1-pound fresh green beans, ends trimmed
- ½ tablespoon olive oil
- ¼ teaspoon salt
- ½ tablespoons fresh dill, minced
- Juice of 1 lemon
- ¼ cup crushed almonds
- Salt as needed

Directions:
- Preheat your oven to 400 °F
- Add in the green beans with your olive oil and also the salt
- Then spread them in one single layer on a large-sized sheet pan
- Roast for 10 minutes and stir nicely, then roast for another 8-10 minutes
- Remove it from the oven and keep stirring in the lemon juice alongside the dill
- Top it with crushed almonds, some flaky sea salt and serve

Nutrition:
Calories: 347
Fat: 16g
Carbohydrates: 6g
Protein: 45g

Cucumber Soup

Preparation Time: 14 minutes
Cooking Time: 0 minutes
Serving: 4

Ingredients:
- 2 tablespoons garlic, minced
- 4 cups English cucumbers, peeled and diced
- ½ cup onions, diced
- tablespoon lemon juice
- ½ cups vegetable broth
- ½ teaspoon salt
- ¼ teaspoon red pepper flakes
- ¼ cup parsley, diced
- ½ cup Greek yogurt, plain

Directions:
- Emulsify all the ingredients by blending them (except ½ cup of chopped cucumbers)
- Blend until smooth
- Divide the soup amongst 4 servings and top with extra cucumbers
- Enjoy chilled!

Nutrition
Calories: 371
Fat: 36g
Carbohydrates: 8g
Protein: 4g

Eggplant Salad

Preparation Time: 10 minutes
Cooking Time: 30 minutes
Serving: 3

Ingredients:
- 2 eggplants, peeled and sliced
- 2 garlic cloves
- 2 green bell paper, sliced, seeds removed
- ½ cup fresh parsley

- ½ cup egg-free mayonnaise
- Salt and black pepper

Directions:
- Preheat your oven to 480 °F
- Take a baking pan and add the eggplants and black pepper
- Bake for about 30 minutes
- Flip the vegetables after 20 minutes
- Then, take a bowl and add baked vegetables and all the remaining ingredients
- Mix well
- Serve and enjoy!

Nutrition:
Calories: 196
Fat: 108.g
Carbohydrates: 13.4g
Protein: 14.6g

Cajun Crab

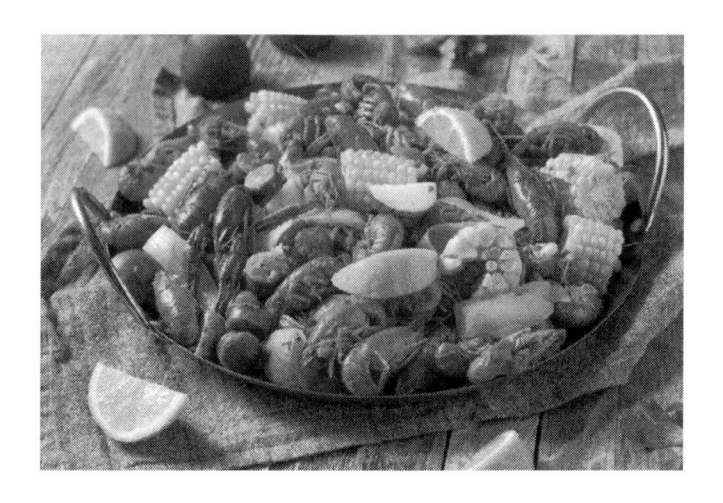

Preparation Time: 10 minutes
Cooking Time: 10 minutes
Serving: 2

Ingredients:
- lemon, fresh and quartered
- tablespoons Cajun seasoning
- bay leaves

- snow crab legs, precooked and defrosted
- Golden ghee

Directions:
- Fill half large pot with salted water about.
- Bring the water to a boil
- Squeeze lemon juice into a pot and toss in remaining lemon quarters
- Add bay leaves and Cajun seasoning
- Then season for 1 minute
- Add crab legs and boil for 8 minutes (make sure to keep them submerged the whole time)
- Melt ghee in the microwave and use as a dipping sauce, enjoy!

Nutrition
Calories: 643
Fat: 51g
Carbohydrates: 3g
Protein: 41g

Mushroom Pork Chops

Preparation Time: 10 minutes
Cooking Time: 40 minutes
Serving: 3

Ingredients:
- 8 ounces mushrooms, sliced
- teaspoon garlic
- onion, peeled and chopped
- cup egg-free mayonnaise
- pork chops, boneless
- teaspoon ground nutmeg
- tablespoon balsamic vinegar
- ½ cup of coconut oil

Directions:
- Take a pan and place it over medium heat
- Add oil and let it heat up
- Add mushrooms, onions, and stir
- Cook for 4 minutes
- Add pork chops, season with nutmeg, garlic powder, and brown both sides
- Transfer the pan in the oven and bake for 30 minutes at 350 °F

- Transfer pork chops to plates and keep it warm
- Take a pan and place it over medium heat
- Add vinegar, mayonnaise over mushroom mix and stir for a few minutes
- Drizzle sauce over pork chops
- Enjoy!

Nutrition:
Calories: 600
Fat: 10g
Carbohydrates: 8g
Protein: 30g

Caramelized Pork Chops

Preparation Time: 5 minutes
Cooking Time: 30 minutes
Serving: 4

Ingredients:
- 4 pounds chuck roast
- 4 ounces green chili, chopped
- 2 tablespoons chili powder
- ½ teaspoon dried oregano
- ½ teaspoon ground cumin
- 2 garlic cloves, minced
- Salt as needed

Directions:
- Rub your chop with 1 teaspoon of pepper and 2 teaspoons of seasoning salt
- Take a skillet and heat some oil over medium heat
- Brown your pork chops on each side
- Add water and onions to the pan
- Simmer it for about 20 minutes
- Turn your chops over and add the rest of the pepper and salt
- Put the lid and cook until there is no water and the onions turn a medium brown texture
- Remove the chops from your pan and serve with some onions on top!

Nutrition
Calories: 271
Fat: 19g
Carbohydrates: 4g
Protein: 27g

Mediterranean Pork

Preparation Time: 10 minutes
Cooking Time: 35 minutes
Serving: 4

Ingredients:
- 4 pork chops, bone-in
- Salt and pepper to taste
- teaspoon dried rosemary
- garlic cloves, peeled and minced

Directions:
- Season pork chops with salt and pepper
- Place in roasting pan
- Add rosemary, garlic in a pan
- Preheat your oven to 425 ° F
- Bake for 10 minutes
- Lower heat to 350 ° F
- Roast for 25 minutes more
- Slice pork and divide on plates
- Drizzle pan juice all over
- Serve and enjoy!

Nutrition:
Calories: 165
Fat: 2g
Carbohydrates: 2g
Protein: 26g

Ground Beef and Bell Peppers

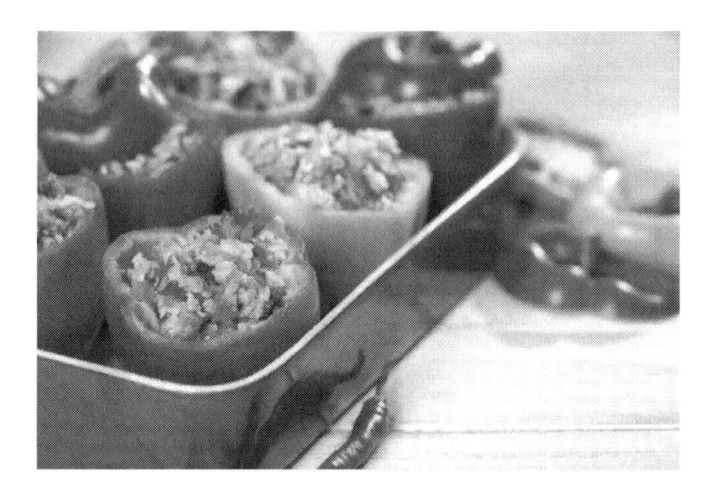

Preparation Time: 10 minutes
Cooking Time: 10 minutes
Serving: 3

Ingredients:
- onion, chopped
- tablespoons coconut oil
- 1-pound ground beef
- red bell pepper, diced
- cups green lettuce, chopped
- Salt and pepper to taste

Directions:
- Place over medium heat on a skillet
- Add onion and cook until slightly browned
- Add green lettuce and ground beef
- Stir fry until done
- Take the mixture and fill up the bell peppers
- Serve and enjoy!

Nutrition
Calories: 350
Fat: 23g
Carbohydrates: 4g
Protein: 28g

Spiced Up Pork Chops

Preparation Time: 4 hours 10 minutes
Cooking Time: 15 minutes
Serving: 4

Ingredients:
- ¼ cup lime juice
- 4 pork rib chops
- tablespoon coconut oil, melted
- garlic cloves, peeled and minced
- tablespoon chili powder
- teaspoon ground cinnamon
- teaspoons cumin
- Salt and pepper to taste
- ½ teaspoon hot pepper sauce
- Mango, sliced

Directions:
- Take a bowl and mix in lime juice, oil, garlic, cumin, cinnamon, chili powder, salt, pepper, hot pepper sauce
- Whisk well
- Add pork chops and toss
- Keep it on the side and refrigerate for 4 hours
- Pre-heat your grill to medium and transfer pork chops to a pre-heated grill
- Grill for 7 minutes both sides
- Divide between serving platters and serve with mango slices
- Enjoy!

Nutrition
Calories: 200
Fat: 8g
Carbohydrates: 3g
Protein: 26g

Juicy Salmon Dish

Preparation Time: 5 minutes
Cooking Time: 6 minutes
Serving: 3

Ingredients:
- ¾ cup of water
- Few sprigs of parsley, basil, tarragon, basil
- pound of salmon, skin on
- teaspoons of ghee
- ¼ teaspoon of salt
- ½ teaspoon of pepper
- ½ of lemon, thinly sliced
- whole carrot, julienned

Directions:
- Set your pot to Sauté mode and add water and herbs
- Place a steamer rack inside your pot and place salmon
- Drizzle ghee on top of the salmon and season with salt and pepper
- Cover with lemon slices
- Cook on HIGH pressure with locked lid for 3 minutes
- Release the pressure naturally over 10 minutes
- Transfer the salmon to a serving platter
- Set your pot to Sauté mode and add vegetables
- Cook for 1-2 minutes
- Serve with vegetables and salmon
- Enjoy!

Nutrition Values
Calories: 464
Fat: 34g
Carbohydrates: 3g
Protein: 34g

Platter-O-Brussels

Preparation Time: 10 minutes
Cooking Time: 20 minutes
Serving: 4

Ingredients:
- 2 tablespoons olive oil
- yellow onion, chopped
- pounds Brussels sprouts, trimmed and halved
- cups chicken stock
- ¼ cup coconut cream

Directions:
- Take a pot and place over medium heat
- Add oil and let it heat up
- Add onion and stir cook for 3 minutes
- Add Brussels sprouts and stir, cook for 2 minutes
- Add stock and black pepper, stir and bring to a simmer
- Cook for 20 minutes more
- Blend until creamy.
- Add coconut cream and stir well
- Ladle into soup bowls and serve
- Enjoy!

Nutrition
Calories: 200
Fat: 11g
Carbohydrates: 6g
Protein: 11g

Almond Chicken

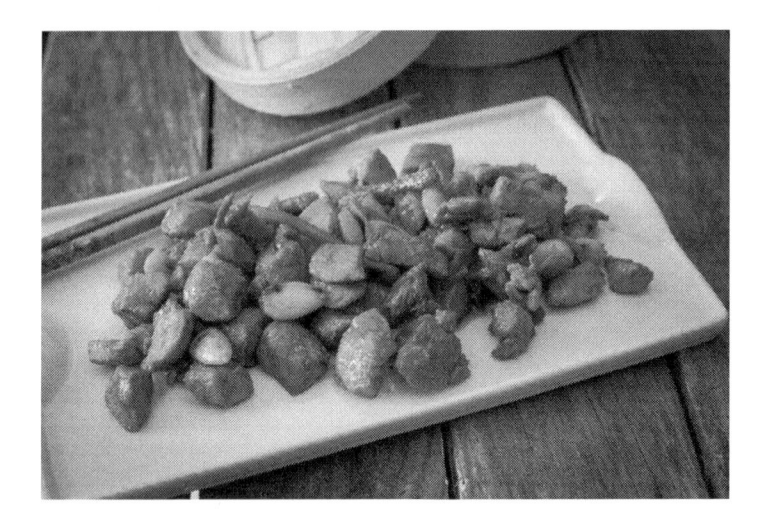

Preparation Time: 15 minutes
Cooking Time: 15 minutes
Serving: 3

Ingredients:
- 2 large chicken breasts, boneless and skinless
- 1/3 cup lemon juice
- ½ cups seasoned almond meal
- tablespoons coconut oil
- Lemon pepper, to taste
- Parsley for decoration

Directions:
- Slice chicken breast in half
- Pound out each half until ¼ inch thick
- Take a pan and place over medium heat, add oil and heat it up
- Dip each chicken breast slice into lemon juice and let it sit for 2 minutes
- Turnover and let the other side sit for 2 minutes as well
- Transfer to almond meal and coat both sides
- Add coated chicken and fry for 4 minutes per side, making sure to sprinkle lemon pepper liberally
- Transfer to a paper-lined sheet and repeat until all chicken is fried
- Garnish with parsley and enjoy!

Nutrition
Calories: 325
Fat: 24g
Carbohydrates: 3g
Protein: 16g

BlackBerry Chicken Wings

Preparation Time: 35 minutes
Cooking Time: 50 minutes
Serving: 4

Ingredients:
- 3 pounds chicken wings, about 20 pieces
- ½ cup blackberry chipotle jam
- Salt and pepper to taste
- ½ cup of water

Directions:
- Add water and jam to a bowl and mix well
- Place chicken wings in a zip bag and add two-thirds of the marinade
- Season with salt and pepper
- Let it marinate for 30 minutes
- Preheat your oven to 400°F
- Prepare a baking sheet and wire rack, place chicken wings in a wire rack and bake for 15 minutes
- Brush remaining marinade and bake for 30 minutes more
- Enjoy!

Nutrition
Calories: 502
Fat: 39g
Carbohydrates: 01.8g
Protein: 34g

Aromatic Carrot Cream

Preparation Time: 15 minutes
Cooking Time: 25 minutes
Servings: 4

Ingredients:
- tablespoon olive oil
- ½ sweet onion, chopped
- teaspoons fresh ginger, peeled and grated
- teaspoon fresh garlic, minced

- cups water
- carrots, chopped
- teaspoon ground turmeric
- ½ cup coconut milk

Directions:
- Heat the olive oil into a big pan over medium-high heat.
- Add the onion, garlic and ginger. Softly cook for about 3 minutes until softened.
- Include the water, turmeric and the carrots. Softly cook for about 20 minutes (until the carrots are softened).
- Blend the soup adding coconut milk until creamy.
- Serve and enjoy!

Nutrition:
Calories 112
Fat 10 g
Cholesterol 0 mg
Carbohydrates 8 g
Sugar 5 g
Fiber 2 g
Protein 2 g
Sodium 35 mg
Calcium 32 mg
Phosphorus 59 mg
Potassium 241 mg

Mushrooms Velvet Soup

Preparation Time: 40 minutes
Cooking Time: 40 minutes
Servings: 6

Ingredients:
- teaspoon olive oil
- ½ teaspoon fresh ground black pepper
- medium (85g) shallots, diced
- stalks (80g) celery, chopped
- clove garlic, diced
- 12-ounces cremini mushrooms, sliced
- tablespoons flour
- cups low sodium vegetable stock, divided

- sprigs fresh thyme
- bay leaves
- ½ cup regular yogurt

Directions:
- Heat oil in a large pan.
- Add ground pepper, shallots and celery. Cook over medium-high heat.
- Sauté for 2 minutes until golden.
- Add garlic and stir.
- Include the sliced mushrooms. Stir and cook until the mushrooms give out their liquid.
- Sprawl the flour on the mushrooms and toast for about 2 min.
- Add one cup of hot stock, thyme sprigs and bay leaves. Stir and add the second cup of stock
- Stir until well combined.
- Add the remaining cups of stock.
- Slowly cook for 15 minutes.
- Take out bay leaves and thyme sprigs.
- Blend until mixture is smooth.
- Include the yogurt and stir well.
- Slowly cook for 4 minutes.
- Serve and enjoy!

Nutrition:
Calories 126
Fat 8 g
Cholesterol 0 mg
Carbohydrate 14 g
Sugar 4 g
Fiber 2 g
Protein 3 g
Sodium 108 mg
Calcium 55 mg
Phosphorus 70 mg
Potassium 298 mg

Easy Lettuce Wraps

Preparation Time: 15 minutes
Cooking Time: 0 minutes
Servings: 4

Ingredients:
- 8 ounces cooked chicken, shredded
- scallion, chopped
- ½ cup seedless red grapes, halved
- celery stalk, chopped
- ¼ cup mayonnaise
- A pinch ground black pepper
- 4 large lettuce leaves

Directions:
- In a mixing bowl add the scallion, chicken, celery, grapes and mayonnaise.
- Stir well until incorporated.
- Season with pepper.
- Place the lettuce leaves onto serving plates.
- Place the chicken salad onto the leaves.
- Serve and enjoy!

Nutrition:
Calories 146
Fat 5 g
Cholesterol 35 mg
Carbohydrates 8 g
Sugar 4 g
Fiber 0 g
Protein 16 g
Sodium 58 mg
Calcium 18 mg
Phosphorus 125 mg
Potassium 212 mg

Spaghetti with Pesto

Preparation Time: 10 minutes
Cooking Time: 10 minutes
Servings: 4

Ingredients:
- 8 ounces spaghetti (package pasta)
- 2 cups packed basil leaves
- 2 cups packed arugula leaves
- 1/3 cup walnut pieces
- 3 cloves of garlic
- ¼ cup extra-virgin olive oil
- Black pepper

Directions:
- Cook pasta with boiling water. Drain.
- Add the basil, garlic, olive oil, walnuts, pepper and arugula in a blender and mix until creamy.
- Mix pesto mixture into pasta in a large bowl.
- Serve and enjoy!

Nutrition:
Calories 400
Fat 21 g
Cholesterol 0 mg
Carbohydrates 46 g
Sugar 2 g
Fiber 3 g
Protein 11 g
Sodium 6 mg
Calcium 64 mg
Phosphorus 113 mg
Potassium 202 mg

Vegetable Casserole

Preparation Time: 15 minutes
Cooking Time: 15 minutes
Servings: 8

Ingredients:
- teaspoon olive oil
- sweet onion, chopped
- teaspoon garlic, minced
- zucchinis, chopped
- red bell pepper, diced
- carrots, chopped
- cups low-sodium vegetable stock
- large Red bell peppers, chopped
- cups broccoli florets
- teaspoon ground coriander
- ½ teaspoon ground comminutes
- Black pepper

Directions:
- Heat the olive oil into a big pan over medium-high heat.
- Add onion and garlic. Softly cook for about 3 minutes until softened.
- Include the zucchini, carrots, bell pepper and softly cook for 5-6 minutes.
- Pour the vegetable stock, Red bell peppers, broccoli, coriander, cumin, pepper and stir well.

- Softly cook for about 5 minutes over medium-high heat until the vegetables are tender.
- Serve hot and enjoy!

Nutrition:
Calories 47
Fat 1 g
Cholesterol 0 g
Carbohydrates 8 g
Sugar 6 g
Fiber 2 g
Protein 2 g
Sodium 104 mg
Calcium 36 mg
Phosphorus 52 mg
Potassium 298 mg

Appetizing Rice Salad

Preparation Time: 20 minutes
Cooking Time: 1 hour
Servings: 8

Ingredients:
- cup wild rice
- cups water
- tablespoon olive oil
- 2/3 cup walnuts, chopped
- (4 inches) celery rib, sliced
- scallions, thinly sliced
- medium red apple, cored and diced
- ½ cup pomegranate seeds
- ½ tablespoon lemon zest
- tablespoons lemon juice
- Black pepper
- 1/3 cup olive oil

Directions:
- In a big pot place the wild strained rice together with water and olive oil.
- Bring to a boil and simmer for about 50 minutes until rice is tender.
- In a mixing bowl add celery, walnuts, apple, scallions, pomegranate seeds and lemon zest.
- Mix well with a blender the lemon juice, pepper, and olive oil.
- Spread half of this dressing on the apple mixture and mix well.
- When the rice is cooked, let it cool and incorporate with the fruit mixture
- Season with the remaining dressing.
- Serve at room temperature and enjoy!

Nutrition:
Calories 300
Fat 19 g
Cholesterol 0 mg
Carbohydrates 34 g
Sugar 11 g
Fiber 5 g
Protein 6 g
Sodium 6 mg
Calcium 30 mg
Phosphorus 144 mg
Potassium 296 mg

Spiced Wraps

Preparation Time: 30 minutes
Cooking Time: 0 minutes
Servings: 8

Ingredients:
- 6 ounces cooked chicken breast, minced
- scallion, chopped
- ½ red apple, cored and chopped
- ½ cup bean sprouts
- ¼ cucumber, chopped
- Juice of 1 lime
- Zest of 1 lime
- tablespoons fresh cilantro, chopped
- ½ teaspoon Chinese five-spice powder
- 8 lettuce leaves

Directions:
- Combine the chicken, apple, bean sprouts, cucumber, lime juice, lime zest, cilantro, five-spice powder and scallions.
- Place the lettuce leaves onto 8 serving plates.
- Spoon the chicken mixture onto lettuce leaves.
- Wrap the lettuce around the chicken mixture.
- Serve and enjoy!

Nutrition:
Calories 53
Fat 3 g
Cholesterol 19 mg
Carbohydrates 3 g
Sugar 3 g
Fiber 2 g
Protein 7 g
Sodium 19 mg
Calcium 16 mg
Phosphorus 58 mg
Potassium 134

Rump Roast

Preparation Time: 10 minutes
Cooking Time: 5 hours
Servings: 8

Ingredients:
- 1-pound rump roast
- ½ teaspoon black pepper
- tablespoon olive oil
- ½ small onion, chopped
- teaspoons garlic, minced
- teaspoon dried thyme
- cup + 3 tablespoons water
- tablespoons cornstarch

Directions:
- Heat the olive oil into a big saucepan over medium heat.
- Add the peppered meat and brown the roast all over. Set aside the meat.
- Softly cook the garlic and onion in the same saucepan for about 3 minutes until they are tendered.
- Incorporate the roast to the saucepan, add 1 cup of water and the thyme.
- Cover, simmer until the meat is tender or for 4 and half hours.
- In a mixing bowl, stir the cornstarch with 3 tablespoons water to form a slurry.
- Beat the slurry into the liquid in the pan and cook for about 15 minutes to thicken the sauce.
- Serve and enjoy!

Nutrition:
Calories 156
Fat 12 g
Cholesterol 42 mg
Carbohydrates 4 g
Sugar 2 g
Fiber 0 g
Protein 14 g
Sodium 48 mg
Calcium 18 mg
Phosphorus 114 mg
Potassium 220 mg

CHAPTER 7:

DINNER

Beef Kabobs with Pepper

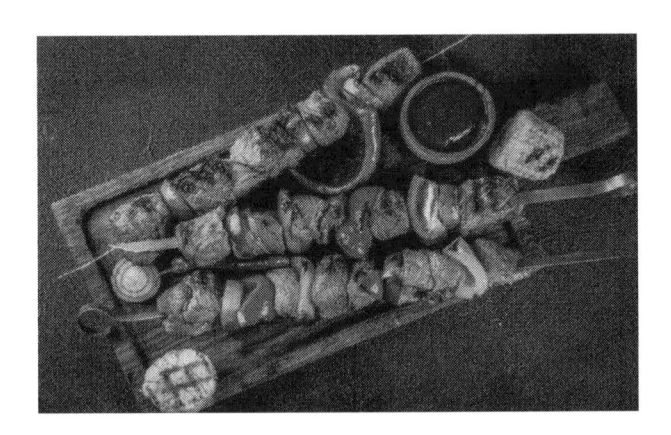

Preparation Time: 5 Minutes
Cooking Time: 10 Minutes
Servings: 8

Ingredients:
- Pound of beef sirloin
- 1/2 Cup of vinegar
- tbsp. of salad oil
- Medium, chopped onion
- tbsp. of chopped fresh parsley
- 1/4 tsp. of black pepper
- Cut into strips green peppers

Directions:
- Trim the fat from the meat; then cut it into cubes of 1 and 1/2 inches each
- Mix the vinegar, the oil, the onion, the parsley and the pepper in a bowl
- Place the meat in the marinade and set it aside for about 2 hours; make sure to stir from time to time.
- Remove the meat from the marinade and alternate it on skewers instead with green pepper
- Brush the pepper with the marinade and broil for about 10 minutes 4 inches from the heat
- Serve and enjoy your kabobs

Nutrition:
Calories: 357 kcal
Total Fat: 24 g
Saturated Fat: 0 g
Cholesterol: 9 mg
Sodium: 60 mg
Total Carbs: 0 g

One-Pot Beef Roast

Preparation Time: 10 minutes
Cooking Time: 75 minutes
Servings: 4

Ingredients:
- 3 1/2 pounds beef roast
- 4 ounces mushrooms, sliced
- 12 ounces beef stock
- 1-ounce onion soup mix
- 1/2 cup Italian dressing

Directions:
- Take a bowl and add the stock, onion soup mix, and Italian dressing
- Stir
- Put beef roast in pan
- Add the mushrooms and stock mix to the pan and cover with foil
- Preheat your oven to 300 °F
- Bake for 1 hour and 15 minutes
- Let the roast cool
- Slice and serve
- Enjoy the gravy on top!

Nutrition:
Calories: 700 kcal
Total Fat: 56 g
Saturated Fat: 0 g
Cholesterol: 0 mg
Sodium: 0 mg
Total Carbs: 10 g

Cabbage and Beef Fry

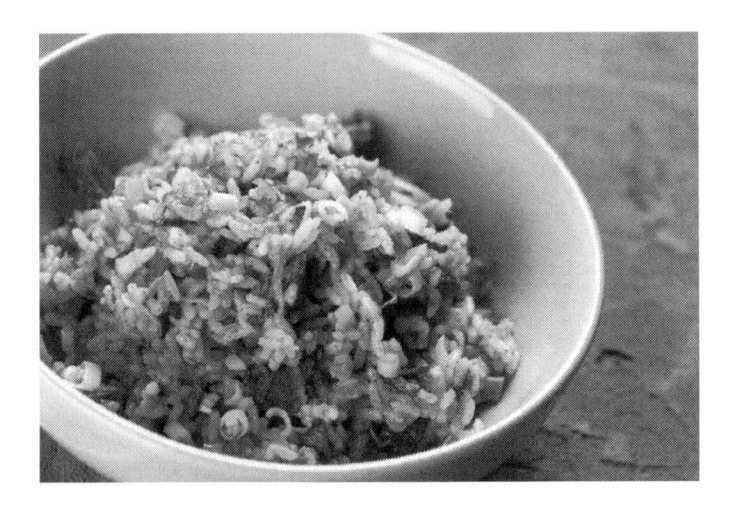

Preparation Time: 5 minutes
Cooking Time: 15 minutes
Servings: 4

Ingredients:
- 1 pound beef, ground
- 1/2 pound bacon
- 1 onion
- 1 garlic cloves, minced
- 1/2 head cabbage
- Salt and pepper to taste

Directions:
- Take a skillet and place it over medium heat
- Add chopped bacon, beef and onion until slightly browned
- Transfer to a bowl and keep it covered
- Add minced garlic and cabbage to the skillet and cook until slightly browned
- Return the ground beef mixture to the skillet and simmer for 3-5 minutes over low heat
- Serve and enjoy!

Nutrition:
Calories: 360 kcal
Total Fat: 22 g
Saturated Fat: 0 g
Cholesterol: 0 mg
Sodium: 0 mg
Total Carbs: 5 g

California Pork Chops

Preparation Time: 10 minutes
Cooking Time: 10 minutes
Servings: 2

Ingredients:
- tbsp. fresh cilantro, chopped
- 1/2 cup chives, chopped
- large green bell peppers, chopped
- lb. 1" thick boneless pork chops
- tbsp. fresh lime juice
- cups cooked rice
- 1/8 tsp. dried oregano leaves
- 1/4 tsp. ground black pepper
- 1/4 tsp. ground cumin
- tbsp. butter
- lime

Directions:
- Start by seasoning the pork chops with lime juice and cilantro.
- Place them in a shallow dish.
- Toss the chives with pepper, cumin, butter, oregano and rice in a bowl.
- Stuff the bell peppers with this mixture and place them around the pork chops.
- Cover the chop and bell peppers with a foil sheet and bake them for 10 minutes in the oven at 375 degrees f.
- Serve warm.

Nutrition:
Calories: 265 kcal
Total Fat: 15 g
Saturated Fat: 0 g
Cholesterol: 86 mg
Sodium: 70 mg
Total Carbs: 24 g
Fiber: 1 g
Sugar: 0 g
Protein: 34 g

Caribbean Turkey Curry

Preparation Time: 10 minutes
Cooking Time: 1 hour an 30 minutes
Servings: 6

Ingredients:
- 3 1/2 lbs. turkey breast, with skin
- 1/4 cup butter, melted
- 1/4 cup honey
- tbsp. mustard
- tsp. curry powder
- tsp. garlic powder

Directions:
- Place the turkey breast in a shallow roasting pan.
- Insert a meat thermometer to monitor the temperature.
- Bake the turkey for 1.5 hours at 350 degrees f until its internal temperature reaches 170 degrees f.
- Meanwhile, thoroughly mix honey, butter, curry powder, garlic powder, and mustard in a bowl.
- Glaze the cooked turkey with this mixture liberally.
- Let it sit for 15 minutes for absorption.
- Slice and serve.

Nutrition:
Calories: 275 kcal
Total Fat: 13 g
Saturated Fat: 0 g
Cholesterol: 82 mg
Sodium: 122 mg
Total Carbs: 90 g

Chicken Fajitas

Preparation Time: 10 minutes
Cooking Time: 10 minutes
Servings: 8

Ingredients:
- 8 flour tortillas, 6" size

- 1/4 cup green pepper, cut in strips
- 1/4 cup red pepper, cut in strips
- 1/2 cup onion, sliced
- 1/2 cup cilantro
- 2 tbsp. canola oil
- 12 oz. boneless chicken breasts
- 1/4 tsp. black pepper
- 2 tsp. chili powder
- 1/2 tsp. cumin
- 2 tbsp. lemon juice

Directions:
- Start by wrapping the tortillas in a foil.
- Warm them up for 10 minutes in a preheated oven at 300 degrees f.
- Add oil to a nonstick pan.
- Add lemon juice chicken and seasoning
- Stir fry for 5 minutes then add onion and peppers.
- Continue cooking for 5 minutes or until chicken is tender.
- Stir in cilantro, mix well and serve in tortillas.

Nutrition:
Calories: 343 kcal
Total Fat: 13 g
Saturated Fat: 0 g
Cholesterol: 53 mg
Sodium: 281 mg
Total Carbs: 33 g

Chicken Veronique

Preparation Time: 10 minutes
Cooking Time: 10 minutes
Servings: 4

Ingredients:
- 2 boneless skinless chicken breasts
- 1/2 shallot, chopped
- 2 tablespoons butter
- 2 tablespoons dry white wine
- 2 tablespoons chicken broth
- 1/2 cup green grapes, halved

- 1 teaspoon dried tarragon
- 1/4 cup cream

Directions:
- Place an 8-inch skillet over medium heat and add butter to melt.
- Sear the chicken in the melted butter until golden-brown on both sides.
- Place the boneless chicken on a plate and set it aside.
- Add shallot to the same skillet and stir until soft.
- Whisk cornstarch with broth and wine in a small bowl.
- Pour this slurry into the skillet and mix well.
- Place the chicken in the skillet and cook it on a simmer for 6 minutes.
- Transfer the chicken to the serving plate.
- Add cream, tarragon, and grapes.
- Cook for 1 minute, and then pour this sauce over the chicken.
- Serve.

Nutrition:
Calories: 306 kcal
Total Fat: 18 g
Saturated Fat: 0 g
Cholesterol: 124 mg
Sodium: 167 mg
Total Carbs: 9 g

Chicken and Apple Curry

Preparation Time: 10 minutes
Cooking Time: 1 hour and 11 minutes
Servings: 8

Ingredients:
- 8 boneless skinless chicken breasts
- 1/4 teaspoon black pepper
- 2 medium apples, peeled, cored, and chopped
- 2 small onions, chopped
- garlic clove, minced
- tablespoons butter
- tablespoon curry powder

- 1/2 tablespoon dried basil
- tablespoons flour
- cup chicken broth
- cup of rice milk

Directions:
- Preheat oven to 350°F.
- Set the chicken breasts in a baking pan and sprinkle black pepper over it.
- Place a suitably-sized saucepan over medium heat and add butter to melt.
- Add onion, garlic, and apple, then sauté until soft.
- Stir in basil and curry powder, and then cook for 1 minute.
- Add flour and continue mixing for 1 minute.
- Stir in rice milk and chicken broth, then stir cook for 5 minutes.
- Pour this sauce over the chicken breasts in the baking pan.
- Bake the chicken for 60 minutes then serve.

Nutrition:
Calories: 232 kcal
Total Fat: 8 g
Saturated Fat: 0 g
Cholesterol: 85 mg
Sodium: 118 mg
Total Carbs: 11 g

London Broil

Preparation Time: 10 minutes
Cooking Time: 5 minutes
Servings: 4

Ingredients:
- 2 pounds flank steak
- 1/4 teaspoon meat tenderizer
- 1 tablespoon sugar
- 2 tablespoons lemon juice
- 2 tablespoons soy sauce
- 1 tablespoon honey
- 1 teaspoon herb seasoning blend

Directions:
- Pound the meat with a mallet then place it in a shallow dish.

- Sprinkle meat tenderizer over the meat.
- Whisk rest of the ingredients and spread this marinade over the meat.
- Marinate the meat for 4 hours in the refrigerator.
- Bake the meat for 5 minutes per side at 350°F.
- Slice and serve.

Nutrition:
Calories: 184 kcal
Total Fat: 8 g
Saturated Fat: 0 g
Cholesterol: 43 mg
Sodium: 208 mg
Total Carbs: 3 g

Sirloin with Squash and Pineapple

Preparation Time: 10 minutes
Cooking Time: 9 minutes
Servings: 2

Ingredients:
- 8 ounces canned pineapple slices
- 2 garlic cloves, minced
- 2 teaspoons ginger root, minced
- 3 teaspoons olive oil
- 1 pound sirloin tips
- 1 medium zucchini, diced
- 1 medium yellow squash, diced
- 1/2 medium red onion, diced

Directions:
- Mix pineapple juice with 1 teaspoon olive oil, ginger, and garlic in a Ziplock bag.
- Add sirloin tips to the pineapple juice marinade and seal the bag.
- Place the bag in the refrigerator overnight.
- Preheat oven to 450°F.
- Layer 2 sheet pans with foil and grease it with 1 teaspoon olive oil.
- Spread the squash, onion, and pineapple rings in the prepared pans.
- Bake them for 5 minutes then transfer to the serving plate.
- Place the marinated sirloin tips on a baking sheet and bake for 4 minutes in the oven.
- Transfer the sirloin tips to the roasted vegetables.

- Serve.

Nutrition:
Calories: 264 kcal
Total Fat: 12 g
Saturated Fat: 0 g
Cholesterol: 74 mg
Sodium: 150 mg
Total Carbs: 14 g

Slow-Cooked BBQ Beef

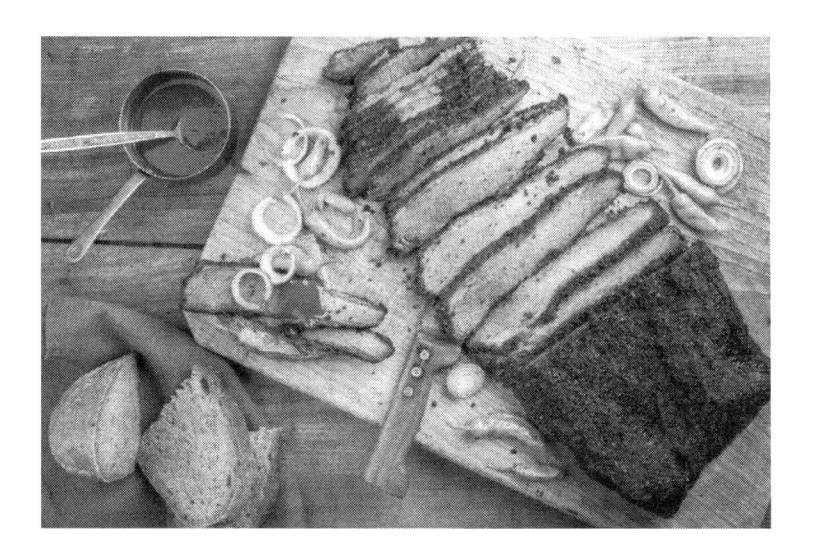

Preparation Time: 10 minutes
Cooking Time: 30 minutes
Servings: 4

Ingredients:
- 4-pound pot roast
- 2 cups of water
- ¾ cup ketchup
- 1/4 cup brown sugar
- 1/3 cup vinegar
- 1/2 teaspoon allspice
- 1/4 cup onion

Directions:
- Add 2 cups water and roast to a Crockpot and cover it.

- Cook for 10 hours on LOW setting, then drain it while keeping 1 cup of its liquid.
- Transfer the cooked meat to a 9x13 pan and set it aside.
- Whisk 1 cup liquid, ketchup, vinegar, brown sugar, minced onion, and allspice in a bowl.
- Add beef to the marinade and mix well to coat, then marinate overnight in the refrigerator.
- Spread it on a baking pan then bake for 30 minutes at 350°F.
- Serve.

Nutrition:
Calories: 303 kcal
Total Fat: 17 g
Saturated Fat: 0 g
Cholesterol: 71 mg
Sodium: 207 mg
Total Carbs: 7 g

Lemon Sprouts

Preparation Time: 10 minutes
Cooking Time: 0
Servings: 4

Ingredients:
- 1 pound Brussels sprouts, trimmed and shredded
- 8 tablespoons olive oil
- 1 lemon, juiced and zested
- Salt and pepper to taste
- ¾ cup spicy almond and seed mix

Directions:
- Take a bowl and mix in lemon juice, salt, pepper and olive oil
- Mix well
- Stir in shredded Brussels sprouts and toss
- Let it sit for 10 minutes
- Add nuts and toss
- Serve and enjoy!

Nutrition:
Calories: 382
Fat: 36g
Carbohydrates: 9g
Protein: 7g

Lemon and Broccoli Platter

Preparation Time: 10 minutes
Cooking Time: 15 minutes
Servings: 6

Ingredients:
- 2 heads broccoli, separated into florets
- 2 teaspoons extra virgin olive oil
- teaspoon salt
- 1/2 teaspoon black pepper
- garlic clove, minced
- 1/2 teaspoon lemon juice

Directions:
- Preheat your oven to 400 °F
- Take a large-sized bowl and add broccoli florets
- Drizzle olive oil and season with pepper, salt, and garlic
- Spread the broccoli out in a single even layer on a baking sheet
- Bake for 15-20 minutes until fork tender
- Squeeze lemon juice on top
- Serve and enjoy!

Nutrition:
Calories: 49
Fat: 1.9g
Carbohydrates: 7g
Protein: 3g

Chicken Liver Stew

Preparation Time: 10 minutes
Cooking Time: 20 minutes
Servings: 2

Ingredients:
- 10 ounces chicken livers
- 1-ounce onion, chopped

- 2 ounces sour cream
- tablespoon olive oil
- Salt to taste

Directions:
- Take a pan and place it over medium heat
- Add oil and let it heat up
- Add onions and fry until just browned
- Add livers and season with salt
- Cook until livers are half cooked
- Transfer the mix to a stew pot
- Add sour cream and cook for 20 minutes
- Serve and enjoy!

Nutrition:
Calories: 146
Fat: 9g
Carbohydrates: 2g
Protein: 15g

Simple Lamb Chops

Preparation Time: 35 minutes
Cooking Time: 5 minutes
Servings: 3

Ingredients:
- 1/4 cup olive oil
- 1/4 cup mint, fresh and chopped
- 8 lamb rib chops
- tablespoon garlic, minced
- tablespoon rosemary, fresh and chopped

Directions:
- Add rosemary, garlic, mint, olive oil into a bowl and mix well
- Keep a tablespoon of the mixture on the side for later use
- Toss lamb chops into the marinade, letting them marinate for 30 minutes
- Take a cast-iron skillet and place it over medium-high heat
- Add lamb and cook for 2 minutes per side for medium-rare
- Let the lamb rest for a few minutes and drizzle the remaining marinade
- Serve and enjoy!

Nutrition:
Calories: 566
Fat: 40g
Carbohydrates: 2g
Protein: 47g

Chicken and Mushroom Stew

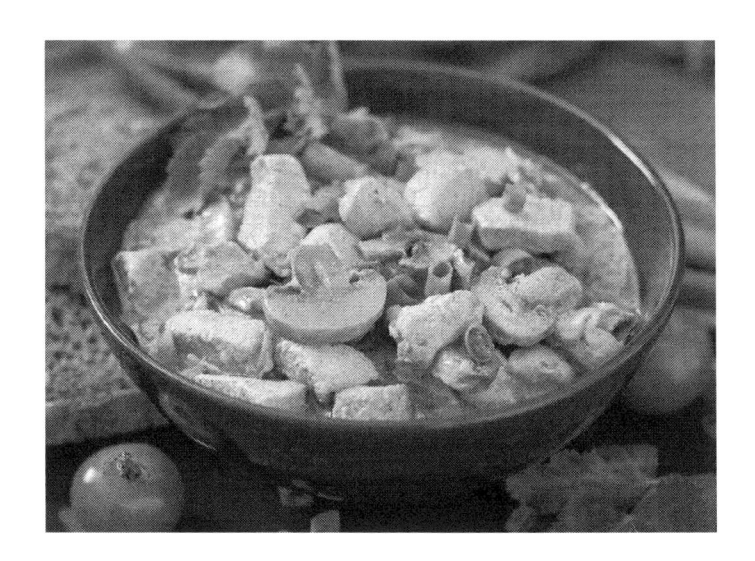

Preparation Time: 10 minutes
Cooking Time: 35 minutes
Servings: 4

Ingredients:
- 4 chicken breast halves, cut into bite-sized pieces
- pound mushrooms, sliced (5-6 cups)
- bunch spring onion, chopped
- 4 tablespoons olive oil
- teaspoon thyme
- Salt and pepper as needed

Directions:
- Take a large deep frying pan and place it over medium-high heat
- Add oil and let it heat up
- Add chicken and cook for 4-5 minutes per side until slightly browned
- Add spring onions and mushrooms, season with salt and pepper according to your taste
- Stir
- Cover with lid and bring the mix to a boil

- Lower heat and simmer for 25 minutes
- Serve!

Nutrition:
Calories: 247
Fat: 12g
Carbohydrates: 10g
Protein: 23g

Roasted Carrot Soup

Preparation Time: 10 minutes
Cooking Time: 50 minutes
Servings: 4

Ingredients:
- 8 large carrots, washed and peeled
- 6 tablespoons olive oil
- 1-quart broth
- Cayenne pepper to taste
- Salt and pepper to taste

Directions:
- Preheat your oven to 425 °F
- Take a baking sheet and add carrots, drizzle olive oil and roast for 30-45 minutes
- Put roasted carrots into a blender and add the broth, puree
- Pour into saucepan and heat soup
- Season with salt, pepper, and cayenne
- Drizzle olive oil
- Serve and enjoy!

Nutrition:
Calories: 222
Fat: 18g
Net Carbohydrates: 7g
Protein: 5g

Garlic and Butter-Flavored Cod

Preparation Time: 5 minutes
Cooking Time: 20 minutes
Servings: 3

Ingredients:

- 3 Cod fillets, 8 ounces each
- ¾ pound baby bok choy halved
- 1/3 cup almond butter, thinly sliced
- 1 1/2 tablespoons garlic, minced
- Salt and pepper to taste

Directions:

- Preheat your oven to 400 °F
- Cut 3 sheets of aluminum foil (large enough to fit fillet)
- Place cod fillet on each sheet and add butter and garlic on top
- Add bok choy, season with pepper and salt
- Fold packet and enclose them in pouches
- Arrange on baking sheet
- Bake for 20 minutes
- Transfer to a cooling rack and let them cool
- Enjoy!

Nutrition:
Calories: 355
Fat: 21g
Carbohydrates: 3g
Protein: 37g

Tilapia Broccoli Platter

Preparation Time: 4 minutes
Cooking Time: 14 minutes
Servings: 2

Ingredients:

- 6 ounces of tilapia, frozen
- 1 tablespoon of almond butter
- 1 tablespoon of garlic, minced
- 1 teaspoon of lemon pepper seasoning
- 1 cup of broccoli florets, fresh

Directions:
- Preheat your oven to 350 °F
- Add fish in aluminum foil packets
- Arrange the broccoli around fish
- Sprinkle lemon pepper on top
- Close the packets and seal
- Bake for 14 minutes
- Take a bowl and add garlic and butter, mix well and keep the mixture on the side
- Remove the packet from the oven and transfer to a platter
- Place butter on top of the fish and broccoli, serve and enjoy!

Nutrition:
Calories: 362
Fat: 25g
Carbohydrates: 2g
Protein: 29g

Parsley Scallops

Preparation Time: 5 minutes
Cooking Time: 25 minutes
Servings: 4

Ingredients:
- 8 tablespoons almond butter
- 2 garlic cloves, minced
- 16 large sea scallops
- Salt and pepper to taste
- 1 1/2 tablespoons olive oil

Directions:
- Seasons scallops with salt and pepper
- Take a skillet and place it over medium heat, add oil and let it heat up
- Sauté scallops for 2 minutes per side, repeat until all scallops are cooked
- Add butter to the skillet and let it melt
- Stir in garlic and cook for 15 minutes
- Return scallops to skillet and stir to coat
- Serve and enjoy!

Nutrition:
Calories: 417

Fat: 31g
Net Carbohydrates: 5g
Protein: 29g

Blackened Chicken

Preparation Time: 10 minutes
Cooking Time: 10 minutes
Servings: 4

Ingredients:
- 1/2 teaspoon paprika
- 1/8 teaspoon salt
- 1/4 teaspoon cayenne pepper
- 1/4 teaspoon ground cumin
- 1/4 teaspoon dried thyme
- 1/8 teaspoon ground white pepper
- 1/8 teaspoon onion powder
- 2 chicken breasts, boneless and skinless

Directions:
- Preheat your oven to 350 °F
- Grease baking sheet
- Take a cast-iron skillet and place it over high heat
- Add oil and heat it up for 5 minutes until smoking hot
- Take a small bowl and mix salt, paprika, cumin, white pepper, cayenne, thyme, onion powder
- Oil the chicken breast on both sides and coat the breast with the spice mix
- Transfer to your hot pan and cook for 1 minute per side
- Transfer to your prepared baking sheet and bake for 5 minutes
- Serve and enjoy!

Nutrition:
Calories: 136
Fat: 3g
Carbohydrates: 1g
Protein: 24g

Spicy Paprika Lamb Chops

Preparation Time: 10 minutes
Cooking Time: 15 minutes
Servings: 4

Ingredients:

- 2 lamb racks, cut into chops
- Salt and pepper to taste
- 3 tablespoons paprika
- ¾ cup cumin powder
- 1 teaspoon chili powder

Directions:

- Take a bowl and add the paprika, cumin, chili, salt, pepper, and stir
- Add lamb chops and rub the mixture
- Heat grill over medium-temperature and add lamb chops, cook for 5 minutes
- Flip and cook for 5 minutes more, flip again
- Cook for 2 minutes, flip and cook for 2 minutes more
- Serve and enjoy!

Nutrition:
Calories: 200
Fat: 5g
Carbohydrates: 4g
Protein: 8g

Mushroom and Olive Sirloin Steak

Preparation Time: 10 minutes
Cooking Time: 14 minutes
Servings: 4

Ingredients:

- 1 pound boneless beef sirloin steak, ¾ inch thick, cut into 4 pieces
- 1 large red onion, chopped
- 1 cup mushrooms
- 4 garlic cloves, thinly sliced
- 4 tablespoons olive oil
- 1 cup parsley leaves, finely cut

Directions:

- Take a large-sized skillet and place it over medium-high heat
- Add oil and let it heat up
- Add beef and cook until both sides are browned, remove beef and drain fat
- Add the rest of the oil to skillet and heat it up
- Add onions, garlic and cook for 2-3 minutes
- Stir well
- Return beef to skillet and lower heat to medium
- Cook for 3-4 minutes (covered)
- Stir in parsley
- Serve and enjoy!

Nutrition:
Calories: 386
Fat: 30g
Carbohydrates: 11g
Protein: 21g

Parsley and Chicken Breast

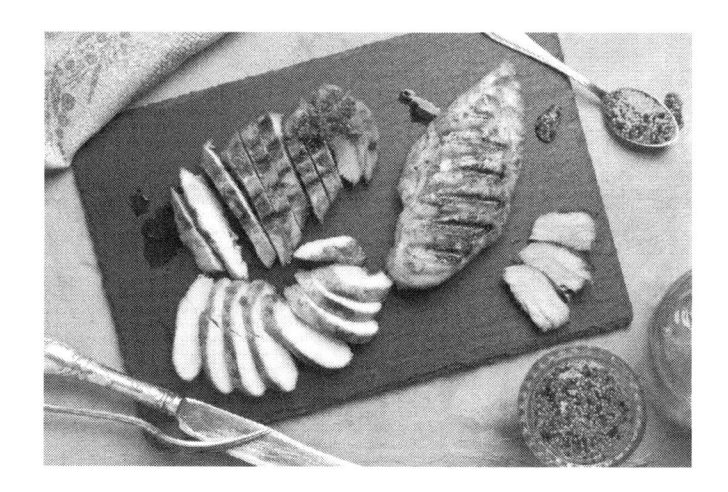

Preparation Time: 10 minutes
Cooking Time: 40 minutes
Servings: 4

Ingredients:

- 1 tablespoon dry parsley
- 1 tablespoon dry basil
- 4 chicken breast halves, boneless and skinless

- 1/2 teaspoon salt
- 1/2 teaspoon red pepper flakes, crushed

Directions:
- Preheat your oven to 350 °F
- Take a 9x13 inch baking dish and grease it with cooking spray
- Sprinkle 1 tablespoon of parsley, 1 teaspoon of basil and spread the mixture over your baking dish
- Arrange the chicken breast halves over the dish and sprinkle garlic slices on top
- Take a small bowl and add 1 teaspoon parsley, 1 teaspoon of basil, salt, basil, red pepper and mix well. Pour the mixture over the chicken breast
- Bake for 25 minutes
- Remove the cover and bake for 15 minutes more
- Serve and enjoy!

Nutrition:
Calories: 150
Fat: 4g
Carbohydrates: 4g
Protein: 25g

Simple Mustard Chicken

Preparation Time: 10 minutes
Cooking Time: 40 minutes
Servings: 4

Ingredients:
- 4 chicken breasts
- 1/2 cup chicken broth
- 3-4 tablespoons mustard
- 3 tablespoons olive oil
- 1 teaspoon paprika
- 1 teaspoon chili powder
- 1 teaspoon garlic powder

Directions:
- Take a small bowl and mix mustard, olive oil, paprika, chicken broth, garlic powder, chicken broth, and chili
- Add chicken breast and marinate for 30 minutes
- Take a lined baking sheet and arrange the chicken

- Bake for 35 minutes at 375 °F
- Serve and enjoy!

Nutrition:
Calories: 531
Fat: 23g
Carbohydrates: 10g
Protein: 64g

Golden Eggplant Fries

Preparation Time: 10 minutes
Cooking Time: 15 minutes
Servings: 8

Ingredients:
- 2 eggs
- 2 cups almond flour
- 2 tablespoons coconut oil, spray
- 2 eggplant, peeled and cut thinly
- Sunflower seeds and pepper

Directions:
- Preheat your oven to 400 degrees F.
- Take a bowl and mix with sunflower seeds and black pepper.
- Take another bowl and beat eggs until frothy.
- Dip the eggplant pieces into the eggs.
- Then coat them with the flour mixture.
- Add another layer of flour and egg.
- Then, take a baking sheet and grease with coconut oil on top.
- Bake for about 15 minutes.
- Serve and enjoy!

Nutrition: Calories: 212
Fat: 15.8g
Carbohydrates: 12.1g
Protein: 8.6g
Phosphorus: 150mg
Potassium: 147mg
Sodium: 105mg

Very Wild Mushroom Pilaf

Preparation Time: 10 minutes
Cooking Time: 3 hours
Servings: 4

Ingredients:
- 1 cup wild rice
- 2 garlic cloves, minced
- 6 green onions, chopped
- 2 tablespoons olive oil
- ½ pound baby Bella mushrooms
- 2 cups water

Directions:
- Add rice, garlic, onion, oil, mushrooms and water to your Slow Cooker.
- Stir well until mixed.
- Place lid and cook on LOW for 3 hours.
- Stir pilaf and divide between serving platters.
- Enjoy!

Nutrition:
Calories: 210
Fat: 7g
Carbohydrates: 16g
Protein: 4g
Phosphorus: 110mg
Potassium: 117mg
Sodium: 75mg

Sporty Baby Carrots

Preparation Time: 5 minutes
Cooking Time: 5 minutes
Servings: 4

Ingredients:
- 1-pound baby carrots
- cup water
- tablespoon clarified ghee
- tablespoon chopped up fresh mint leaves
- Sea flavored vinegar as needed

Directions:
- Place a steamer rack on top of your pot and add the carrots.
- Add water.
- Lock the lid and cook at HIGH pressure for 2 minutes.
- Do a quick release.
- Pass the carrots through a strainer and drain them.
- Wipe the insert clean.
- Return the insert to the pot and set the pot to Sauté mode.
- Add clarified butter and allow it to melt.
- Add mint and sauté for 30 seconds.
- Add carrots to the insert and sauté well.
- Remove them and sprinkle with bit of flavored vinegar on top.
- Enjoy!

Nutrition: Calories: 131 Fat: 10g Carbohydrates: 11g Protein: 1g Phosphorus: 130mg Potassium: 147mg Sodium: 85mg

Saucy Garlic Greens

Preparation Time: 5 minutes
Cooking Time: 20 minutes
Servings: 4

Ingredients:
- bunch of leafy greens
- Sauce
- ½ cup cashews soaked in water for 10 minutes
- ¼ cup water
- tablespoon lemon juice
- teaspoon coconut aminos
- clove peeled whole clove
- 1/8 teaspoon of flavored vinegar

Directions:

- Make the sauce by draining and discarding the soaking water from your cashews and add the cashews to a blender.
- Add fresh water, lemon juice, flavored vinegar, coconut aminos, and garlic.
- Blitz until you have a smooth cream and transfer to bowl.
- Add ½ cup of water to the pot.
- Place the steamer basket to the pot and add the greens in the basket.
- Lock the lid and steam for 1 minute.
- Quick-release the pressure.
- Transfer the steamed greens to strainer and extract excess water.

- Place the greens into a mixing bowl.
- Add lemon garlic sauce and toss.
- Enjoy!

Nutrition:
Calories: 77
Fat: 5g
Carbohydrates: 0g
Protein: 2g
Phosphorus: 120mg
Potassium: 137mg
Sodium: 85mg

Garden Salad

Preparation Time: 5 minutes
Cooking Time: 20 minutes
Servings: 6

Ingredients:
- 1-pound raw peanuts in shell
- 1 bay leaf
- 2 medium-sized chopped up Red bell peppers
- ½ cup diced up green pepper
- ½ cup diced up sweet onion
- ¼ cup finely diced hot pepper
- ¼ cup diced up celery
- 2 tablespoons olive oil
- ¾ teaspoon flavored vinegar
- ¼ teaspoon freshly ground black pepper

Directions:
- Boil your peanuts for 1 minute and rinse them.
- The skin will be soft, so discard the skin.
- Add 2 cups of water to the Instant Pot.
- Add bay leaf and peanuts.
- Lock the lid and cook on HIGH pressure for 20 minutes.
- Drain the water.

- Take a large bowl and add the peanuts, diced up vegetables.
- Whisk in olive oil, lemon juice, pepper in another bowl.
- Pour the mixture over the salad and mix.
- Enjoy!

Nutrition:
Calories: 140
Fat: 4g
Carbohydrates: 24g
Protein: 5g
Phosphorus: 110mg
Potassium: 117mg
Sodium: 75mg

Spicy Cabbage Dish

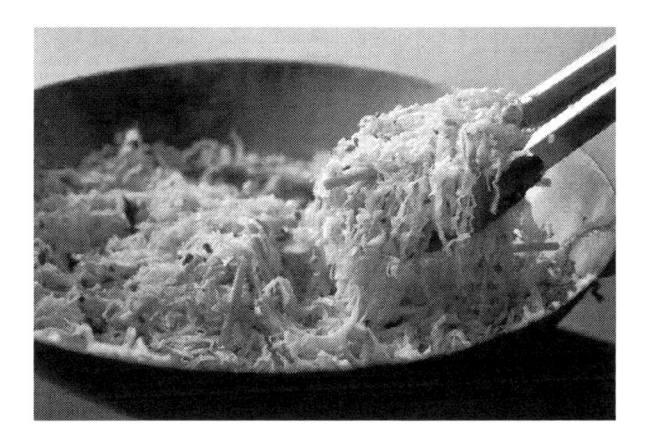

Preparation Time: 10 minutes
Cooking Time: 4 hours
Servings: 4

Ingredients:
- 2 yellow onions, chopped
- 10 cups red cabbage, shredded
- 1 cup plums, pitted and chopped
- 1 teaspoon cinnamon powder
- 1 garlic clove, minced
- 1 teaspoon cumin seeds
- ¼ teaspoon cloves, ground
- 2 tablespoons red wine vinegar
- 1 teaspoon coriander seeds
- ½ cup water

Directions:
- Add cabbage, onion, plums, garlic, cumin, cinnamon, cloves, vinegar, coriander and water to your Slow Cooker.
- Stir well.
- Place lid and cook on LOW for 4 hours.
- Divide between serving platters.
- Enjoy!

Nutrition:
Calories: 197
Fat: 1g
Carbohydrates: 14g
Protein: 3g
Phosphorus: 115mg
Potassium: 119mg
Sodium: 75mg

Extreme Balsamic Chicken

Preparation Time: 10 minutes
Cooking Time: 35 minutes
Servings: 4

Ingredients:
- 3 boneless chicken breasts, skinless
- Sunflower seeds to taste
- ¼ cup almond flour
- 2/3 cups low-fat chicken broth
- 1 ½ teaspoons arrowroot

- ½ cup low sugar raspberry preserve
- 1 ½ tablespoons balsamic vinegar

Directions:
- Cut chicken breast into bite-sized pieces and season them with seeds.
- Dredge the chicken pieces in flour and shake off any excess.
- Take a non-stick skillet and place it over medium heat.
- Add chicken to the skillet and cook for 15 minutes, making sure to turn them half-way through.
- Remove chicken and transfer to platter.
- Add arrowroot, broth, raspberry preserve to the skillet and stir.
- Stir in balsamic vinegar and reduce heat to low, stir-cook for a few minutes.
- Transfer the chicken back to the sauce and cook for 15 minutes more.
- Serve and enjoy!

Nutrition: Calories: 546 Fat: 35g Carbohydrates: 11g Protein: 44g Phosphorus: 120mg Potassium: 117mg Sodium: 85mg

Enjoyable Green lettuce and Bean Medley

Servings: 4
Preparation Time: 10 minutes
Cooking Time: 4 hours

Ingredients:
- 5 carrots, sliced
- 1 ½ cups great northern beans, dried
- 2 garlic cloves, minced
- 1 yellow onion, chopped
- Pepper to taste
- ½ teaspoon oregano, dried
- 5 ounces baby green lettuce
- 4 ½ cups low sodium veggie stock
- 2 teaspoons lemon peel, grated
- 3 tablespoon lemon juice

Directions:
- Add beans, onion, carrots, garlic, oregano and stock to your Slow Cooker.
- Stir well.
- Place lid and cook on HIGH for 4 hours.
- Add green lettuce, lemon juice and lemon peel.
- Stir and let it sit for 5 minutes.

- Divide between serving platters and enjoy!

Nutrition: Calories: 219 Fat: 8g Carbohydrates: 14g Protein: 8g Phosphorus: 210mg Potassium: 217mg Sodium: 85mg

Tantalizing Cauliflower and Dill Mash

Preparation Time: 10 minutes
Cooking Time: 6 hours
Servings: 6

Ingredients:
- 1 cauliflower head, florets separated
- 1/3 cup dill, chopped
- 6 garlic cloves
- 2 tablespoons olive oil
- Pinch of black pepper

Directions:
- Add cauliflower to Slow Cooker.
- Add dill, garlic and water to cover them.
- Place lid and cook on HIGH for 5 hours.
- Drain the flowers.
- Season with pepper and add oil, mash using potato masher.
- Whisk and serve.
- Enjoy!

Nutrition: Calories: 207 Fat: 4g Carbohydrates: 14g Protein: 3g Phosphorus: 130mg Potassium: 107mg Sodium: 105mg

Peas Soup

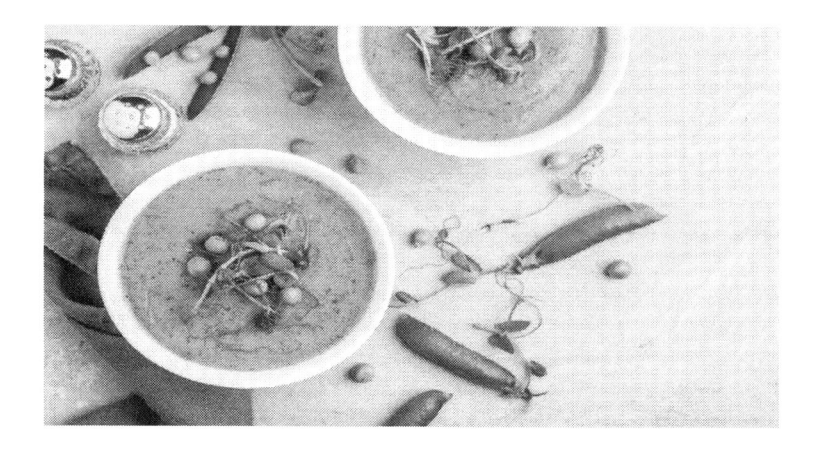

Preparation Time: 10 minutes
Cooking Time: 10 minutes
Servings: 4

Ingredients:
- 1 white onion, chopped
- 1 quart veggie stock
- 2 eggs
- 3 tablespoons lemon juice
- 2 cups peas
- 2 tablespoons parmesan, grated
- Salt and black pepper to the taste

Directions:
- Heat up a pot with the oil over medium-high heat, add the onion and sauté for 4 minutes.
- Add the rest of the ingredients except the eggs, bring to a simmer and cook for 4 minutes.
- Add whisked eggs, stir the soup, cook for 2 minutes more, divide into bowls and serve.

Nutrition:
Calories 293,
fat 11.2
fiber 3.4,
carbs 27,
protein 4.45

Minty Lamb Stew

Preparation Time: 10 minutes
Cooking Time: 1 hour and 45 minutes
Servings: 4

Ingredients:
- ½ cup mint, chopped
- Salt and black pepper to the taste
- 2 pounds lamb shoulder, boneless and cubed
- 3 tablespoons oil
- 1 carrot, chopped
- 1 yellow onion, chopped
- 1 celery rib, chopped
- 1 tablespoon ginger, grated
- 1 tablespoon garlic, minced
- ½ cup mint, chopped
- 15 ounces canned chickpeas, drained
- 6 tablespoons Greek yogurt

Directions:
- Heat up a pot with 2 tablespoons oil over medium-high heat, add the meat and brown for 5 minutes.
- Add the carrot, onion, celery, garlic and the ginger, stir and sauté for 5 minutes more.
- Add the rest of the ingredients except the yogurt, bring to a simmer and cook over medium heat for 1 hour and 30 minutes.
- Divide the stew into bowls, top each serving with the yogurt and serve.

Nutrition: Calories 355, fat 14.3, fiber 6.7, carbs 22.6, protein 15.4

Spicy Mushroom Stir-Fry

Preparation Time: 10 minutes
Cooking Time: 10 minutes
Servings: 4

Ingredients:
- 1 cup low-sodium vegetable broth
- 2 tablespoons cornstarch
- 1 teaspoon low-sodium soy sauce
- 1/2 teaspoon ground ginger

- 1/8 teaspoon cayenne pepper
- 2 tablespoons olive oil
- 2 (8-ounce) packages sliced button mushrooms
- 1 red bell pepper, chopped
- 1 jalapeño pepper, minced
- 2 tablespoons sesame oil

Directions:
- In a small bowl, whisk together the broth, cornstarch, soy sauce, ginger, and cayenne pepper and set aside.
- Heat the olive oil in a wok or heavy skillet over high heat.
- Add the mushrooms and peppers and stir-fry for 3 to 5 minutes or until the vegetables are tender-crisp.
- Stir the broth mixture and add it to the wok; stir-fry for 3 to 5 minutes longer or until the vegetables are tender and the sauce has thickened.
- Serve

Nutrition:
Calories: 361
Fat: 16g
Carbohydrates: 49g
Protein: 8g
Sodium: 95mg
Phosphorus: 267mg
Potassium: 582mg

Curried Veggies and Rice

Preparation Time: 12 minutes
Cooking Time: 18 minutes
Servings: 4

Ingredients:
- 1/4 cup olive oil
- 1 cup long-grain white basmati rice
- 4 garlic cloves, minced
- 2 1/2 teaspoons curry powder
- 1/2 cup sliced shiitake mushrooms
- 1 red bell pepper, chopped
- 1 cup frozen, shelled edamame
- 2 cups low-sodium vegetable broth
- 1/8 teaspoon freshly ground black pepper

Directions:
- Heat the olive oil on medium heat.
- Add the rice, garlic, curry powder, mushrooms, bell pepper, and edamame; cook, stirring, for 2 minutes.
- Add the broth and black pepper and bring to a boil.
- Reduce the heat to low, partially cover the pot, and simmer for 15 to 18 minutes or until the rice is tender. Stir and serve.

Nutrition:
Calories: 347
Fat: 16g
Carbohydrates: 44g
Protein: 8g
Sodium: 114mg
Phosphorus: 131mg
Potassium: 334mg

Spicy Veggie Pancakes

Preparation Time: 10 minutes
Cooking Time: 10 minutes
Servings: 4

Ingredients:
- 3 tablespoons olive oil, divided
- 2 small onions, finely chopped
- 1 jalapeño pepper, minced
- 3/4 cup carrot, grated
- 3/4 cup cabbage, finely chopped
- 1 1/2 cups quick-cooking oats
- 3/4 cup of water
- ½ cup whole-wheat flour
- 1 large egg
- 1 large egg white
- 1 teaspoon baking soda
- 1/4 teaspoon cayenne pepper

Directions:
- In a skillet, heat 2 teaspoons oil over medium heat.
- Sauté the onion, jalapeño, carrot, and cabbage for 4 minutes.
- While the veggies are cooking, combine the oats, rice, water, flour, egg, egg white, baking soda, and cayenne pepper in a medium bowl until well mixed.
- Add the cooked vegetables to the mixture and stir to combine.
- Heat the remaining oil in a large skillet over medium heat.
- Drop the mixture into the skillet, about 1/3 cup per pancake. Cook for 4 minutes, or until bubbles form on the pancakes' surface and the edges look cooked, then carefully flip them over.
- Repeat with the remaining mixture and serve.

Nutrition:
Calories: 323
Fat: 11g
Carbohydrates: 48g
Protein: 10g
Sodium: 366mg
Potassium: 381mg
Phosphorus: 263mg

Egg and Veggie Fajitas

Preparation Time: 15 minutes
Cooking Time: 10 minutes
Servings: 4

Ingredients:
- 3 large eggs
- 3 egg whites
- 2 teaspoons chili powder
- 1 tablespoon unsalted butter
- 1 onion, chopped
- 2 garlic cloves, minced
- 1 jalapeño pepper, minced
- 1 red bell pepper, chopped
- 1 cup frozen corn, thawed and drained
- 8 (6-inch) corn tortillas

Directions:
- Whisk the eggs, egg whites, and chili powder in a small bowl until well combined. Set aside.
- Prepare a large skillet and melt the butter on medium heat.
- Sauté the onion, garlic, jalapeño, bell pepper, and corn until the vegetables are tender, 3 to 4 minutes.
- Add the beaten egg mixture to the skillet. Cook, occasionally stirring, until the eggs form large curds and are set, 3 to 5 minutes.
- Meanwhile, soften the corn tortillas as directed on the package.
- Divide the egg mixture evenly among the softened corn tortillas. Roll the tortillas up and serve.

Nutrition:
Calories: 316
Fat 14g
Carbohydrates: 35g
Protein: 14g
Sodium: 167mg
Potassium: 408mg
Phosphorus: 287mg

Vegetable Biryani

Preparation Time: 10 minutes
Cooking Time: 15 minutes
Servings: 4

Ingredients:
- 2 tablespoons olive oil
- 1 onion, diced
- 4 garlic cloves, minced
- 1 tbsp. peeled and grated fresh ginger root
- 1 cup carrot, grated
- 2 cups chopped cauliflower
- 1 cup thawed frozen baby peas
- 2 teaspoons curry powder
- 1 cup low-sodium vegetable broth
- 3 cups of frozen cooked white rice

Directions:
- Get a skillet and heat the olive oil on medium heat.
- Add onion, garlic, and ginger root. Sauté, frequently stirring, until tender-crisp, 2 minutes.
- Add the carrot, cauliflower, peas, and curry powder and cook for 2 minutes longer.
- Put vegetable broth. Cover the skillet partially, and simmer on low for 6 to 7 minutes or until the vegetables are tender.
- Meanwhile, heat the rice as directed on the package.
- Stir the rice into the vegetable mixture and serve.

Nutrition:
Calories: 378
Fat 16g
Carbohydrates: 53g
Protein: 8g
Sodium: 113mg
Potassium: 510mg
Phosphorus: 236mg

Creamy Tuna Salad

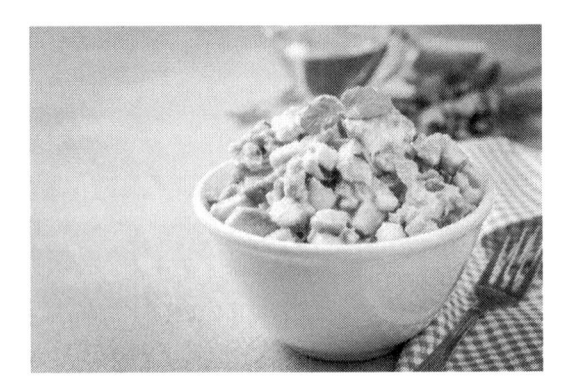

Preparation Time: 10 minutes
Cooking Time: 5 minutes
Servings: 4

Ingredients:
- 3.5 oz. can tuna, drained and flaked
- 1 1/2 tsp garlic powder
- 1 tbsp. dill, chopped
- 1 tsp curry powder
- 2 tbsp. fresh lemon juice
- 1/2 cup onion, chopped
- 1/2 cup celery, chopped
- 1/4 cup parmesan cheese, grated
- 3/4 cup mayonnaise

Directions:
- Add all ingredients into the large bowl and mix until well combined.
- Serve and enjoy.

Nutrition:
Calories 224
Fat 15.5 g
Carbohydrates 14.1 g
Sugar 4.2 g
Protein 8 g
Cholesterol 20 mg
Phosphorus: 110mg
Potassium: 117mg
Sodium: 75mg

Creamy Mushroom Soup

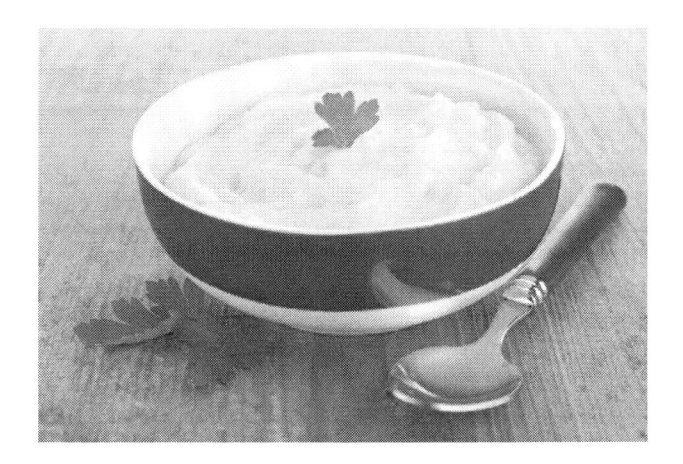

Preparation Time: 10 minutes
Cooking Time: 15 minutes
Servings: 6

Ingredients:
- 1 lb. mushrooms, sliced
- 1/2 cup heavy cream
- 4 cups chicken broth
- 1 tbsp. sage, chopped
- 1/4 cup butter
- Pepper
- Salt

Directions:
- Melt butter in a large pot over medium heat.
- Add sage and saute for 1 minute.
- Add mushrooms and cook for 3-5 minutes or until lightly browned.
- Add broth and stir well and simmer for 5 minutes.
- Puree the soup using an immersion blender until smooth.
- Add heavy cream and stir well. Season soup with pepper and salt.
- Serve hot and enjoy.

Nutrition:
Calories 145
Fat 12.5 g
Carbohydrates 3.6 g
Sugar 1.8 g
Protein 5.9 g
Cholesterol 34 mg

Phosphorus: 140mg
Potassium: 127mg
Sodium: 75mg

Pork Soup

Preparation Time: 10 minutes
Cooking Time: 4 hours 15 minutes
Servings: 8

Ingredients:
- 2 lbs. country pork ribs, boneless and cut into 1-inch pieces
- 2 cups cauliflower rice
- 1 1/2 tbsp. fresh oregano, chopped
- 1 cup of water
- 2 cups Red bell peppers, chopped
- 1 cup chicken stock
- 1/2 cup dry white wine
- 1 onion, chopped
- 3 garlic cloves, chopped
- 1 tbsp. olive oil
- Pepper
- Salt

Directions:
- Heat oil in a saucepan over medium heat.
- Season pork with pepper and salt. Add pork into the saucepan and cook until lightly brown from all the sides.
- Add onion and garlic and saute for 2 minutes.
- Add Red bell peppers, water, stock, and white wine and stir well. Bring to boil.
- Pour saucepan mixture into the slow cooker.
- Cover and cook on high for 4 hours.
- Add cauliflower rice and oregano in the last 20 minutes of cooking.
- Stir well and serve.

Nutrition:
Calories 263
Fat 15.1 g
Carbohydrates 5.8 g
Sugar 2.6 g
Protein 23.4 g
Cholesterol 85 mg

Phosphorus: 130mg
Potassium: 117mg
Sodium: 105mg

Thai Chicken Soup

Preparation Time: 10 minutes
Cooking Time: 30 minutes
Servings: 6

Ingredients:
- 4 chicken breasts, slice into 1/4-inch strips
- 1 tbsp. fresh basil, chopped
- 1 tsp ground ginger
- 1 oz. fresh lime juice
- 1 tbsp. coconut aminos
- 2 tbsp. chili garlic paste
- 1/4 cup fish sauce
- 28 oz. water
- 14 oz. chicken broth
- 14 oz. coconut milk

Directions:
- Add coconut milk, basil, ginger, lime juice, coconut aminos, chili garlic paste, fish sauce, water, and broth into the stockpot. Stir well and bring to boil over medium-high heat.
- Add chicken and stir well. Turn heat to medium-low and simmer for 30 minutes.
- Stir well and serve.

Nutrition: Calories 357 Fat 23.4 g Carbohydrates 5.5 g Sugar 2.9 g Protein 31.7 g Cholesterol 87 mg Phosphorus: 110mg Potassium: 117mg Sodium: 75mg

Tasty Pumpkin Soup

Preparation Time: 10 minutes
Cooking Time: 30 minutes
Servings: 6

Ingredients:
- 2 cups pumpkin puree
- 1 cup coconut cream
- 4 cups vegetable broth
- 1/2 tsp ground ginger
- 1 tsp curry powder
- 2 shallots, chopped
- 1/2 onion, chopped
- 4 tbsp. butter
- Pepper
- Salt

Directions:
- Melt butter in a saucepan over medium heat.
- Add shallots and onion and sauté until softened.
- Add ginger and curry powder and stir well.
- Add broth, pumpkin puree, and coconut cream and stir well. Simmer for 10 minutes.
- Puree the soup using an immersion blender until smooth.
- Season with pepper and salt.
- Serve and enjoy.

Nutrition: Calories 229 Fat 18.4 g Carbohydrates 13 g Sugar 4.9 g Protein 5.6 g Cholesterol 20 mg Phosphorus: 120mg Potassium: 137mg Sodium: 95mg

Easy Zucchini Soup

Preparation Time: 10 minutes
Cooking Time: 25 minutes
Servings: 4

Ingredients:
- 5 zucchinis, sliced
- 8 oz. cream cheese, softened
- 5 cups vegetable stock
- Pepper
- Salt

Directions:
- Add zucchini and stock into the stockpot and bring to boil over high heat.
- Turn heat to medium and simmer for 20 minutes.

- Add cream cheese and stir until cheese is melted.
- Puree soup using an immersion blender until smooth.
- Season with pepper and salt.
- Serve and enjoy.

Nutrition: Calories 245 Fat 20.3 g Carbohydrates 10.9 g Sugar 5.2 g Protein 7.7 g Cholesterol 62 mg Phosphorus: 110mg Potassium: 117mg Sodium: 75mg

Quick Tomato Soup

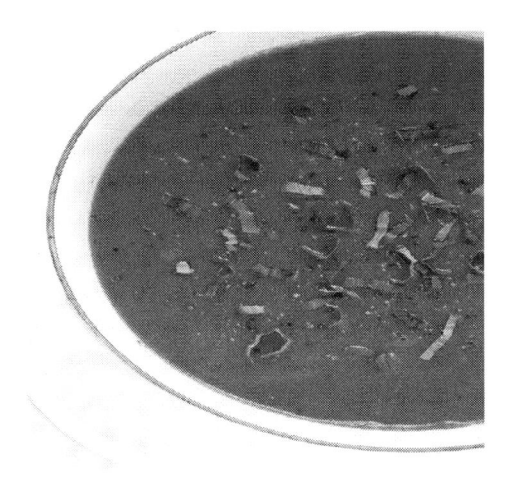

Preparation Time: 10 minutes
Cooking Time: 5 minutes
Servings: 4

Ingredients:
- 28 oz. can tomato, diced
- 1 tbsp. balsamic vinegar
- 1 tbsp. dried basil
- 1 tbsp. dried oregano
- 1 tsp garlic, minced
- 2 tbsp. olive oil
- Pepper
- Salt

Directions:
- Heat oil in a saucepan over medium heat.
- Add basil, oregano, and garlic and saute for 30 seconds.
- Add Red bell peppers, vinegar, pepper, and salt and simmer for 3 minutes.
- Stir well and serve hot.

Nutrition:
Calories 108
Fat 7.1 g
Carbohydrates 11.2 g
Sugar 6.8 g
Protein 2 g
Cholesterol 0 mg
Phosphorus: 130mg
Potassium: 127mg
Sodium: 75mg

Spicy Chicken Soup

Preparation Time: 10 minutes
Cooking Time: 5 minutes
Servings: 4

Ingredients:

- 2 cups cooked chicken, shredded
- 1/2 cup half and half
- 4 cups chicken broth
- 1/3 cup hot sauce
- 3 tbsp. butter
- 4 oz. cream cheese
- Pepper
- Salt

Directions:

- Add half and half, broth, hot sauce, butter, and cream cheese into the blender and blend until smooth.
- Pour blended mixture into the saucepan and cook over medium heat until just hot.
- Add chicken stir well. Season soup with pepper and salt.
- Serve and enjoy.

Nutrition: Calories 361 Fat 25.6 g Carbohydrates 3.3 g Sugar 1.1 g Protein 28.4 g Cholesterol 119 mg Phosphorus: 110mg Potassium: 117mg Sodium: 75mg

Shredded Pork Soup

Preparation Time: 10 minutes
Cooking Time: 8 hours
Servings: 8

Ingredients:
- 1 lb. pork loin
- 8 cups chicken broth
- 2 tsp fresh lime juice
- 1 1/2 tsp garlic powder
- 1 1/2 tsp onion powder
- 1 1/2 tsp chili powder
- 1 1/2 tsp cumin
- 1 jalapeno pepper, minced
- 1 cup onion, chopped
- 3 Red bell peppers, chopped

Directions:
- Add Red bell peppers, jalapeno, and onion into the slow cooker and stir well.
- Place meat on top of the tomato mixture.
- Pour remaining ingredients on top of the meat.
- Cover slow cooker and cook on low for 8 hours.
- Remove meat from slow cooker and shred using a fork.
- Return shredded meat to the slow cooker and stir well.
- Serve and enjoy.

Nutrition: Calories 199 Fat 9.6 g Carbohydrates 6.3 g Sugar 3.1 g Protein 21.2 g Cholesterol 45 mg Phosphorus: 140mg Potassium: 127mg Sodium: 95mg

Creamy Chicken Green lettuce Soup

Preparation Time: 10 minutes
Cooking Time: 10 minutes
Servings: 6

Ingredients:
- 3 cups cooked chicken, shredded
- 1/8 tsp nutmeg
- 4 cup chicken broth

- 1/2 cup parmesan cheese, shredded
- 8 oz. cream cheese
- 1/4 cup butter
- 4 cup baby green lettuce, chopped
- 1 tsp garlic, minced
- Pepper
- Salt

Directions:
- Melt butter in a saucepan over medium heat.
- Add green lettuce and garlic and cook until green lettuce is wilted.
- Add parmesan cheese and cream cheese and stir until cheese is melted.
- Add remaining ingredients and stir everything well and cook for 5 minutes.
- Season soup with pepper and salt.
- Serve and enjoy.

Nutrition: Calories 361 Fat 25.6 g Carbohydrates 2.8 g Sugar 0.6 g Protein 29.5 g Cholesterol 121 mg Phosphorus: 110mg Potassium: 117mg Sodium: 75mg

Shrimp Paella

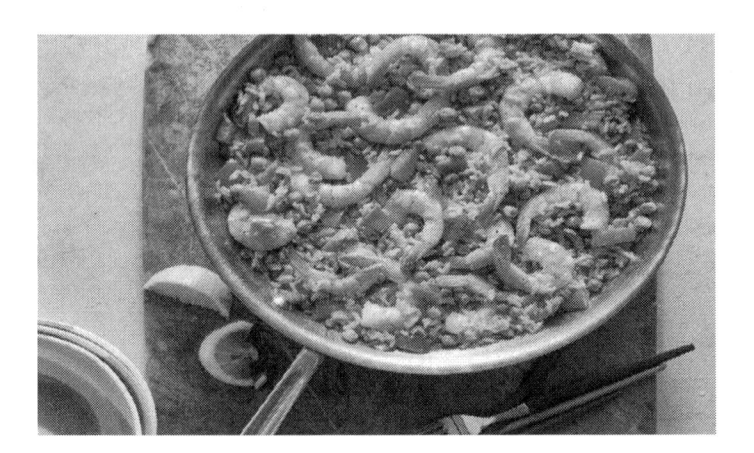

Preparation Time: 5 minutes
Cooking Time: 10 minutes
Servings: 2

Ingredients:
- 1 cup cooked white rice
- 1 chopped red onion
- 1 tsp. paprika

- 1 chopped garlic clove
- 1 tbsp. olive oil
- 6 oz. frozen cooked shrimp
- 1 deseeded and sliced chili pepper
- 1 tbsp. oregano

Directions:
- Warm-up olive oil in a large pan on medium-high heat. Add the onion and garlic and sauté for 2-3 minutes until soft. Now add the shrimp and sauté for a further 5 minutes or until hot through.
- Now add the herbs, spices, chili, and rice with 1/2 cup boiling water. Stir until everything is warm, and the water has been absorbed. Plate up and serve.

Nutrition:
Calories 221
Protein 17 g
Carbs 31 g
Fat 8 g
Sodium 235 mg
Potassium 176 mg
Phosphorus 189 mg

Salmon & Pesto Salad

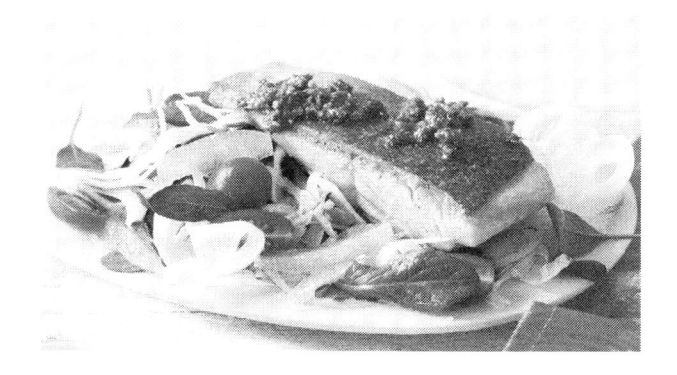

Preparation Time: 5 minutes
Cooking Time: 15 minutes
Servings: 2

Ingredients:
For the pesto:
- minced garlic clove

- ½ cup fresh arugula
- ¼ cup extra virgin olive oil
- ½ cup fresh basil
- tsp black pepper

For the salmon:
- 4 oz. skinless salmon fillet
- tbsp. coconut oil

For the salad:
- ½ juiced lemon
- 2 sliced radishes
- ½ cup iceberg lettuce
- tsp black pepper

Directions:
- Prepare the pesto by blending all the fixing for the pesto in a food processor or grinding with a pestle and mortar. Set aside.
- Add a skillet to the stove on medium-high heat and melt the coconut oil. Add the salmon to the pan. Cook for 7-8 minutes and turn over.
- Cook within 3-4 minutes or until cooked through. Remove fillets from the skillet and allow to rest.
- Mix the lettuce and the radishes and squeeze over the juice of ½ lemon. Shred the salmon using a fork and mix through the salad. Toss to coat and sprinkle with a little black pepper to serve.

Nutrition:
Calories 221
Protein 13 g
Carbs 1 g
Fat 34 g
Sodium 80 mg
Potassium 119 mg
Phosphorus 158 mg

Baked Fennel & Garlic Sea Bass

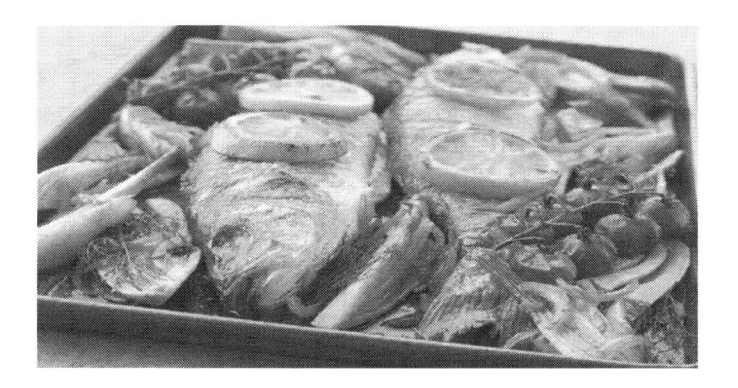

Preparation Time: 5 minutes
Cooking Time: 15 minutes
Servings: 2

Ingredients:
- 1 lemon
- ½ sliced fennel bulb
- 6 oz. sea bass fillets
- 1 tsp black pepper
- 2 garlic cloves

Directions:
- Preheat the oven to 375°F. Sprinkle black pepper over the Sea Bass. Slice the fennel bulb and garlic cloves. Add 1 salmon fillet and half the fennel and garlic to one sheet of baking paper or tin foil.
- Squeeze in 1/2 lemon juices. Repeat for the other fillet. Fold and add to the oven for 12-15 minutes or until fish is thoroughly cooked through.
- Meanwhile, add boiling water to your couscous, cover, and allow to steam. Serve with your choice of rice or salad.

Nutrition:
Calories 221
Protein 14 g
Carbs 3 g
Fat 2 g
Sodium 119 mg
Potassium 398 mg
Phosphorus 149 mg

Lemon, Garlic, Cilantro Tuna and Rice

Preparation Time: 5 minutes
Cooking Time: 0 minutes
Servings: 2

Ingredients:
- ½ cup arugula
- 1 tbsp. extra virgin olive oil
- 1 cup cooked rice
- 1 tsp black pepper
- ¼ finely diced red onion
- 1 juiced lemon
- 3 oz. canned tuna
- 2 tbsp. Chopped fresh cilantro

Directions:
- Mix the olive oil, pepper, cilantro, and red onion in a bowl. Stir in the tuna, cover, then serve with the cooked rice and arugula!

Nutrition:
Calories 221
Protein 11 g
Carbs 26 g
Fat 7 g
Sodium 143 mg
Potassium 197 mg
Phosphorus 182 mg

Cod & Green Bean Risotto

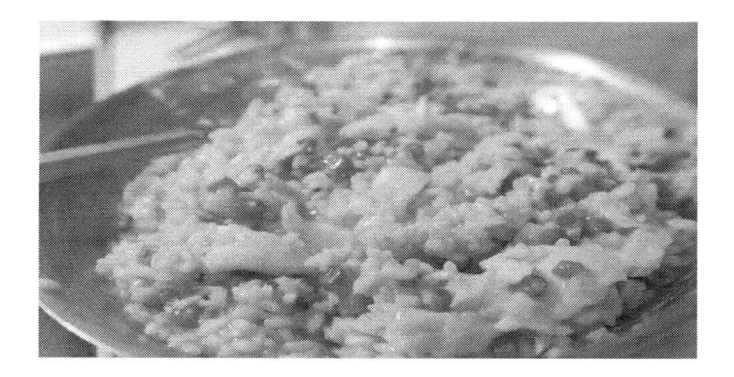

Preparation Time: 4 minutes
Cooking Time: 40 minutes
Servings: 2

Ingredients:
- ½ cup arugula
- finely diced white onion
- 4 oz. cod fillet
- cup white rice
- lemon wedges
- cup boiling water
- ¼ tsp. black pepper
- cup low-sodium chicken broth
- tbsp. extra virgin olive oil
- ½ cup green beans

Directions:
- Warm-up oil in a large pan on medium heat. Sauté the chopped onion for 5 minutes until soft before adding in the rice and stirring for 1-2 minutes.
- Combine the broth with boiling water. Add half of the liquid to the pan and stir. Slowly add the rest of the liquid while continuously stirring for up to 20-30 minutes.
- Stir in the green beans to the risotto. Place the fish on top of the rice, cover, and steam for 10 minutes.
- Use your fork to break up the fish fillets and stir into the rice. Sprinkle with freshly ground pepper to serve and a squeeze of fresh lemon. Serve with the lemon wedges and the arugula.

Nutrition:
Calories 221
Protein 12 g
Carbs 29 g
Fat 8 g

Sodium 398 mg
Potassium 347 mg
Phosphorus 241 mg

Sardine Fish Cakes

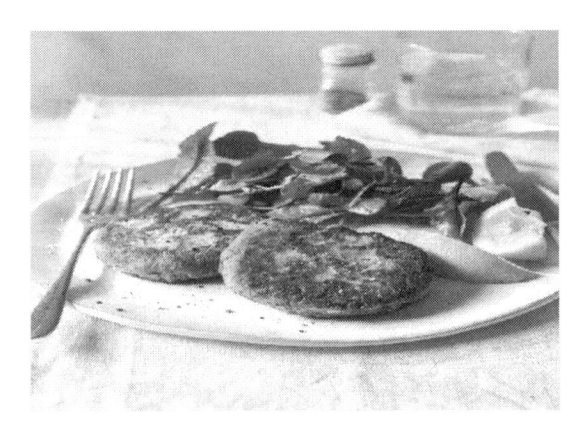

Preparation Time: 10 minutes
Cooking Time: 10 minutes
Servings: 4

Ingredients:
- 11 oz. sardines, canned, drained
- 1/3 cup shallot, chopped
- 1 teaspoon chili flakes
- ½ teaspoon salt
- 2 tablespoon wheat flour, whole grain
- 1 egg, beaten
- 1 tablespoon chives, chopped
- 1 teaspoon olive oil
- 1 teaspoon butter

Directions:
- Put the butter in your skillet and dissolve it. Add shallot and cook it until translucent. After this, transfer the shallot to the mixing bowl.
- Add sardines, chili flakes, salt, flour, egg, chives, and mix up until smooth with the fork's help. Make the medium size cakes and place them in the skillet. Add olive oil.
- Roast the fish cakes for 3 minutes from each side over medium heat. Dry the cooked fish cakes with a paper towel if needed and transfer to the serving plates.

Nutrition:
Calories 221

Fat 12.2g
Fiber 0.1g
Carbs 5.4g
Protein 21.3 g
Phosphorus 188.7 mg
Potassium 160.3 mg
Sodium 452.6 mg

4-Ingredients Salmon Fillet

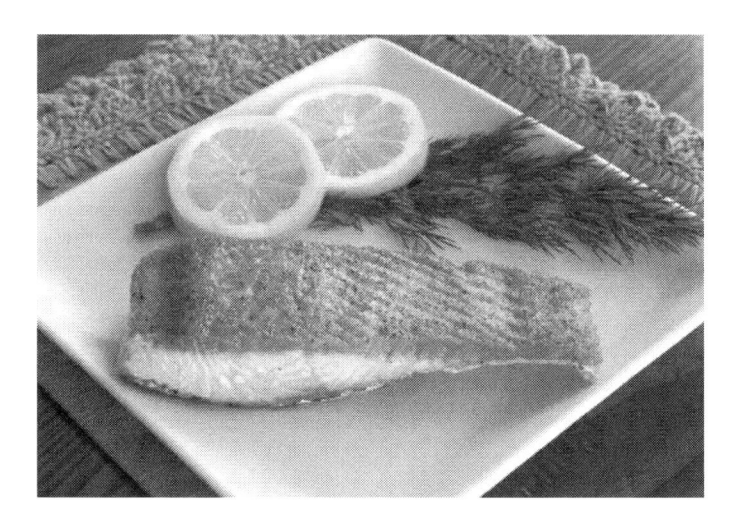

Preparation Time: 5 minutes
Cooking Time: 25 minutes
 Servings: 1

Ingredients:
- 4 oz. salmon fillet
- ½ teaspoon salt
- 1 teaspoon sesame oil
- ½ teaspoon sage

Directions:
- Rub the fillet with salt and sage. Put the fish in the tray, then sprinkle it with sesame oil. Cook the fish for 25 minutes at 365F. Flip the fish carefully onto another side after 12 minutes of cooking. Serve.

Nutrition:
Calories 191

Fat 11.6g
Fiber 0.1g
Carbs 0.2g
Protein 22g
Sodium 70.5 mg
Phosphorus 472 mg
Potassium 636.3 mg

Spanish Cod in Sauce

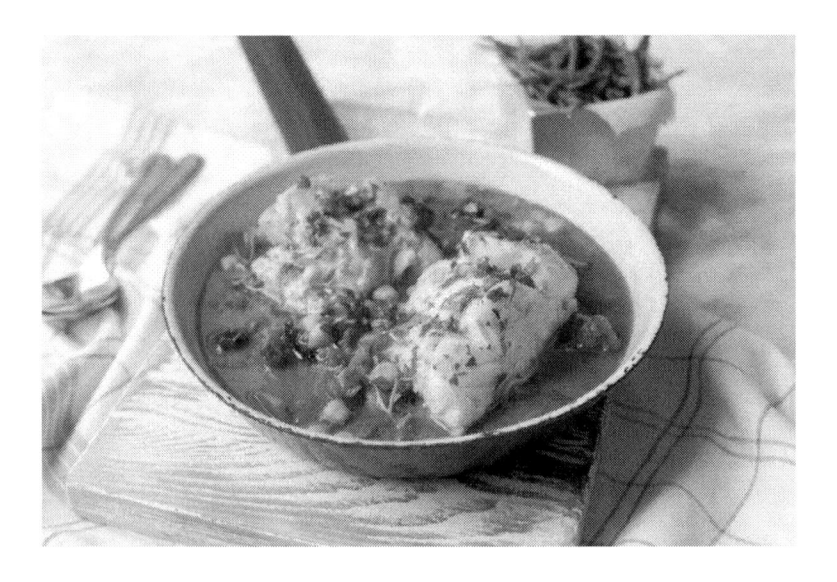

Preparation Time: 10 minutes
Cooking Time: 5 1/2 hours
Servings: 2

Ingredients:
- 1 teaspoon tomato paste
- 1 teaspoon garlic, diced
- 1 white onion, sliced
- 1 jalapeno pepper, chopped
- 1/3 cup chicken stock
- 7 oz. Spanish cod fillet
- 1 teaspoon paprika
- 1 teaspoon salt

Directions:
- Pour chicken stock into the saucepan. Add tomato paste and mix up the liquid until homogenous. Add garlic, onion, jalapeno pepper, paprika, and salt.
- Bring the liquid to boil and then simmer it. Chop the cod fillet and add it to the tomato liquid. Simmer the fish for 10 minutes over low heat. Serve the fish in the bowls with tomato sauce.

Nutrition:
Calories 113
Fat 1.2g
Fiber 1.9g
Carbs 7.2g
Protein 18.9g
Potassium 659 mg
Sodium 597 mg
Phosphorus 18 mg

Salmon Baked in Foil with Fresh Thyme

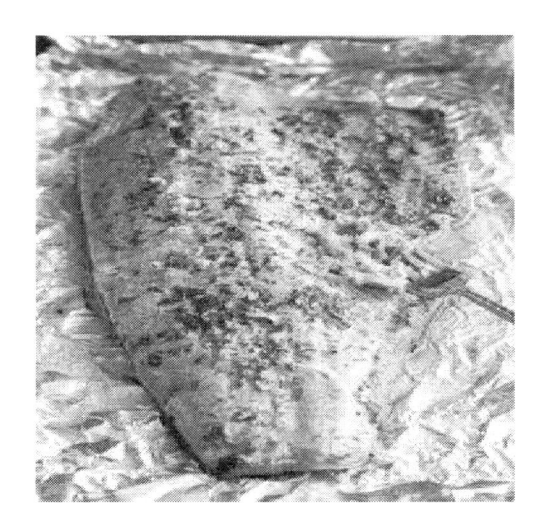

Preparation Time: 10 minutes
Cooking Time: 30 minutes
Servings: 4

Ingredients:
- 4 fresh thyme sprigs
- 4 garlic cloves, peeled, roughly chopped
- 16 oz. salmon fillets (4 oz. each fillet)
- ½ teaspoon salt
- ½ teaspoon ground black pepper

- 4 tablespoons cream
- 4 teaspoons butter
- ¼ teaspoon cumin seeds

Directions:
- Line the baking tray with foil. Sprinkle the fish fillets with salt, ground black pepper, cumin seeds, and arrange them in the tray with oil.
- Add thyme sprig on the top of every fillet. Then add cream, butter, and garlic. Bake the fish for 30 minutes at 345F. Serve.

Nutrition:
Calories 198
Fat 11.6g
Carbs 1.8g
Protein 22.4g
Phosphorus 425 mg
Potassium 660.9 mg
Sodium 366 mg

Poached Halibut in Orange Sauce

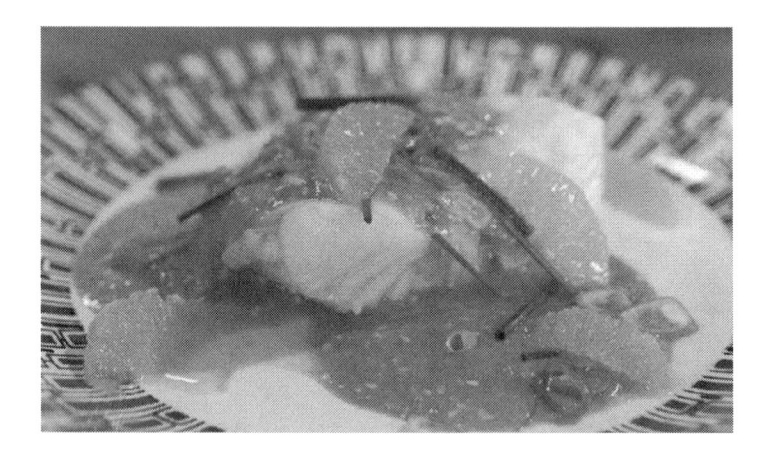

Preparation Time: 10 minutes
Cooking Time: 10 minutes
Servings: 4

Ingredients:
- 1-pound halibut
- 1/3 cup butter
- 1 rosemary sprig

- ½ teaspoon ground black pepper
- 1 teaspoon salt
- 1 teaspoon honey
- ¼ cup of orange juice
- 1 teaspoon cornstarch

Directions:
- Put butter in the saucepan and melt it. Add rosemary sprig. Sprinkle the halibut with salt and ground black pepper. Put the fish in the boiling butter and poach it for 4 minutes.
- Meanwhile, pour orange juice into the skillet. Add honey and bring the liquid to boil. Add cornstarch and whisk until the liquid starts to be thick. Then remove it from the heat.
- Transfer the poached halibut to the plate and cut it on 4. Place every fish serving in the serving plate and top with orange sauce.

Nutrition:
Calories 349
Fat 29.3g
Fiber 0.1g
Carbs 3.2g
Protein 17.8g
Phosphorus 154 mg
Potassium 388.6 mg
Sodium 29.3 mg

CHAPTER 8:

SNACK RECIPES

Veggie Snack

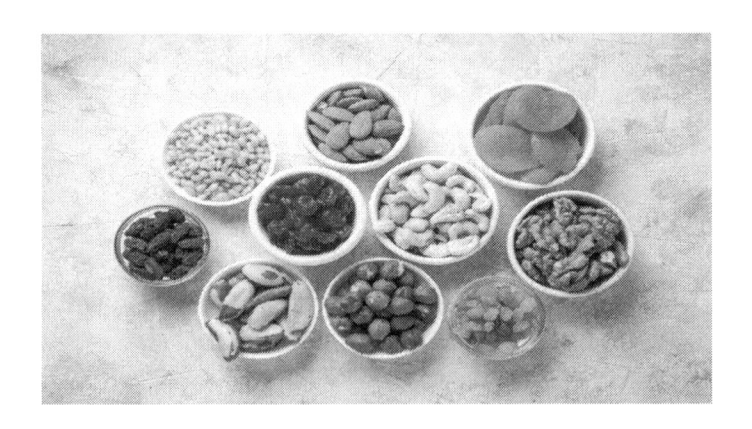

Preparation Time: 5 minutes
Cooking Time: 10 minutes
Servings: 1

Ingredients:
- 1 large yellow pepper
- 5 carrots
- 5 stalks celery

Directions:
- Clean the carrots and rinse under running water.
- Rinse celery and yellow pepper. Remove seeds of pepper and chop the veggies into small sticks.
- Put in a bowl and serve.

Nutrition:
Calories: 189
Fat: 0.5 g
Carbs: 44.3 g
Protein: 5 g
Sodium: 282 mg
Potassium: 0mg
Phosphorus: 0mg

Healthy Spiced Nuts

Preparation Time: 10 minutes
Cooking Time: 10 minutes
Servings: 4

Ingredients:
- 1 tbsp. extra virgin olive oil
- ¼ cup walnuts
- ¼ cup pecans
- ¼ cup almonds
- ½ tsp. sea salt
- ½ tsp. cumin
- ½ tsp. pepper
- 1 tsp. chili powder

Directions:
- Put the skillet on medium heat and toast the nuts until lightly browned.
- Prepare the spice mixture and add black pepper, cumin, chili, and salt.
- Put extra virgin olive oil and sprinkle with spice mixture to the toasted nuts before serving.

Nutrition:
Calories: 88
Fat: 8g
Carbs: 4g
Protein: 2.5g
Sodium: 51mg
Potassium: 88mg
Phosphorus: 6.3mg

Roasted Asparagus

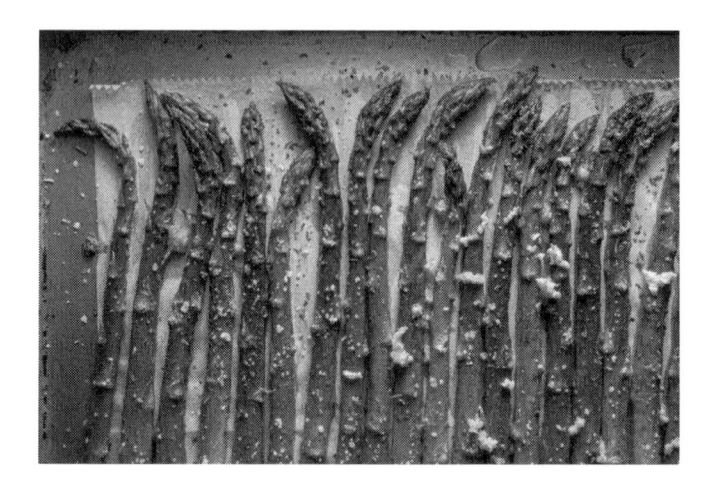

Preparation Time: 5 minutes
Cooking Time: 10 minutes
Servings: 4

Ingredients:
- 1 tbsp. extra virgin olive oil
- 1-pound fresh asparagus
- 1 medium lemon, zested
- 1/2 tsp. freshly grated nutmeg
- 1/2 tsp. kosher salt
- ½ tsp. black pepper

Directions:
- Preheat your oven to 500 degrees F.
- Put asparagus on an aluminum foil and add extra virgin olive oil.
- Prepare asparagus in a single layer and fold the edges of the foil.
- Cook in the oven for 5 minutes. Continue roasting until browned.
- Add the roasted asparagus with nutmeg, salt, zest, and pepper before serving.

Nutrition:
Calories: 55
Fat: 3.8 g
Carbs: 4.7 g
Protein: 2.5 g
Sodium: 98mg
Potassium: 172mg
Phosphorus: 35mg

Low-Fat Mango Salsa

Preparation Time: 10 minutes
Cooking Time: 10 minutes
Servings: 4

Ingredients:
- 1 cup cucumber, chopped
- 2 cups mango, diced
- ½ cup cilantro, minced
- 2 tablespoons fresh lime juice
- 1 tablespoon scallions, minced
- ¼ teaspoon chipotle powder
- ¼ teaspoon sea salt

Directions
- Mix the ingredients in a bowl and serve or refrigerate.

Nutrition:
Calories: 155
Fat: 0.6 g
Carbs: 38.2 g
Protein: 1.4 g
Sodium: 3.2 mg
Potassium: 221mg
Phosphorus: 27mg

Vinegar & Salt Kale

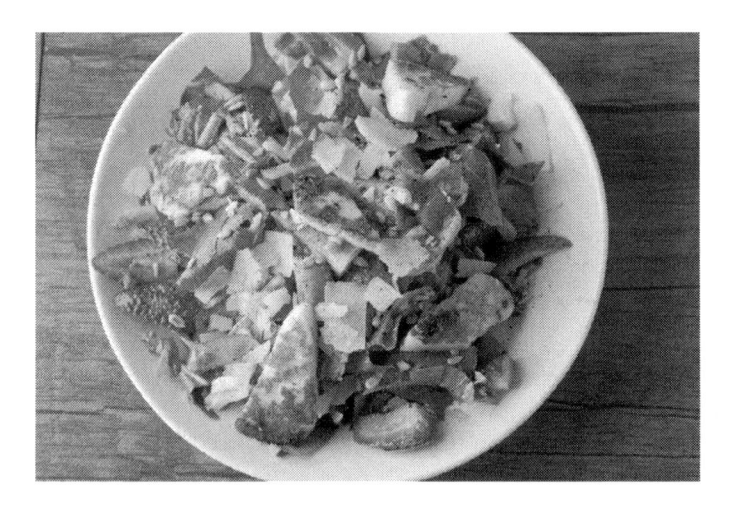

Preparation Time: 10 minutes
Cooking Time: 12 minutes
Servings: 2

Ingredients:
- 1 head kale, chopped
- 1 teaspoon extra virgin olive oil
- 1 tablespoon apple cider vinegar
- ½ teaspoon of sea salt

Directions:
- Prepare kale in a bowl and put vinegar and extra virgin olive oil.
- Sprinkle with salt and massage the ingredients with hands.
- Spread the kale out onto two paper-lined baking sheets and bake at 375°F for about 12 minutes or until crispy.
- Let cool for about 10 minutes before serving.

Nutrition:
Calories: 152
Fat: 8.2 g
Carbs: 15.2 g
Protein: 4 g
Sodium: 170mg
Potassium: 304mg
Phosphorus: 37mg

Carrot and Parsnips French Fries

Preparation Time: 15 minutes
Cooking Time: 20 minutes
Servings: 2

Ingredients:
- 6 large carrots
- 6 large parsnips
- 2 tablespoons extra virgin olive oil
- ½ teaspoon of sea salt

Directions:
- Chop the carrots and parsnips into 2-inch slices and then cut each into thin sticks.
- Toss together the carrots and parsnip sticks with extra virgin olive oil and salt in a bowl and spread into a baking sheet lined with parchment paper.
- Bake the sticks at 425° for about 20 minutes or until browned.

Nutrition:
Calories: 179
Fat: 4g
Carbs: 14g
Protein: 11g
Sodium: 27.3mg
Potassium: 625mg
Phosphorus: 116mg

Apple & Strawberry Snack

Preparation Time: 5 minutes
Cooking Time: 2 minutes
Servings: 1

Ingredients:
- ½ apple, cored and sliced
- 2-3 strawberries
- dash of ground cinnamon
- 2-3 drops stevia 2-3 drops

Directions:
- In a bowl, mix strawberries and apples and sprinkle with stevia and cinnamon.
- Microwave for about 1-2 minutes. Serve warm.

Nutrition:
Calories: 145
Fat: 0.8 g
Carbs: 34.2 g
Protein: 1.6 g
Sodium: 20 mg
Potassium: 0mg
Phosphorus: 0mg

Candied Macadamia Nuts

Preparation Time: 5 minutes
Cooking Time: 15 minutes
Servings: 2

Ingredients:
- 2 cups macadamia nuts
- tablespoon extra-virgin olive oil
- tablespoons honey

Directions:
- Toss ingredients in bowl and spread into a baking dish.
- Bake for 15 minutes at 350°F.
- Let cool before serving.

Nutrition:
Calories: 200
Fat: 18 g
Carbs: 10g
Protein: 1g
Sodium: 5 mg
Potassium: 55mg
Phosphorus: 10mg

Cinnamon Apple Fries

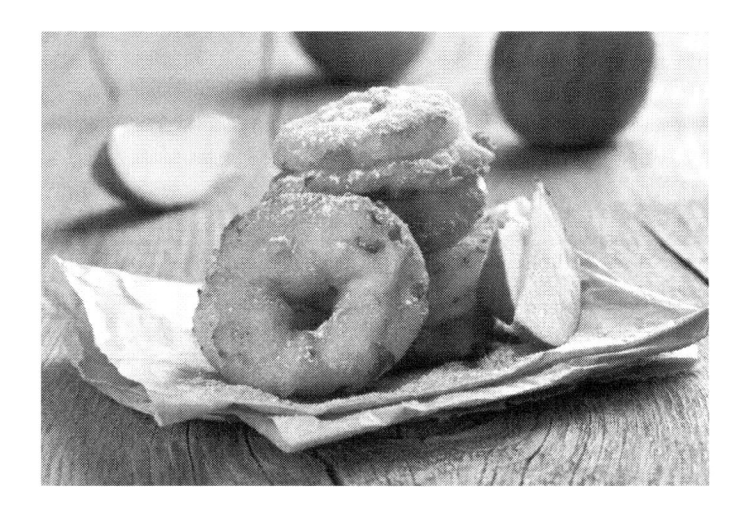

Preparation Time: 5 minutes
Cooking Time: 15 minutes
Servings: 1

Ingredients:
- apple, sliced thinly
- Dash of cinnamon
- Stevia

Directions:
- Coat apple slices with cinnamon and stevia.
- Bake for 15 minutes or until tender and crispy at 325 degrees F.

Nutrition:
Calories: 146
Fat: 0.7 g
Carbs: 36.4 g
Protein: 1.6 g
Sodium: 10 mg
Potassium: 100mg
Phosphorus: 0mg

Lemon Pops

Preparation Time: 5 minutes
Cooking Time: 5 minutes
Servings: 1

Ingredients:
- 4 tablespoons fresh lemon juice
- Powdered stevia

Directions:
- Mix orange or lemon juice and stevia and pour into molds.
- Freeze until firm.

Nutrition:
Calories: 46
Fat: 0.2g
Carbs: 16g
Protein: 0.9g
Sodium: 3.7mg
Potassium: 104mg
Phosphorus: 11mg

Easy No-Bake Coconut Cookies

Preparation Time: 5 minutes
Cooking Time: 10 minutes
Servings: 20

Ingredients:
- 3 cups finely shredded coconut flakes
- 1 cup melted coconut oil
- 1 teaspoon liquid stevia

Directions:
- Prepare all ingredients in a large bowl; stir until well blended.
- Form the mixture into small balls and arrange them on a paper-lined baking tray.
- Press each cookie down with a fork and refrigerate until firm. Enjoy!

Nutrition:
Calories: 99
Fat: 10 g
Carbs: 2 g
Protein: 3 g
Sodium: 7 mg
Potassium: 105mg
Phosphorus: 11mg

Roasted Chili-Vinegar Peanuts

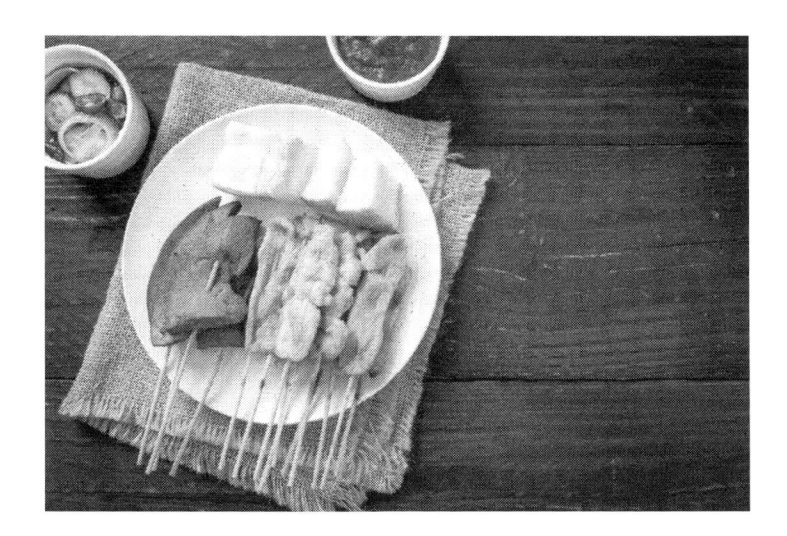

Preparation Time: 5 minutes
Cooking Time: 10 minutes
Servings: 4

Ingredients:
- 1 tablespoon coconut oil
- 2 cups raw peanuts, unsalted
- 2 teaspoon sea salt
- 2 tablespoon apple cider vinegar
- 1 teaspoon chili powder
- 1 teaspoon fresh lime zest

Directions:
- Preheat oven to 350°F.
- In a large bowl, toss together coconut oil, peanuts, and salt until well coated.
- Transfer to a rimmed baking sheet and roast in the oven for about 15 minutes or until fragrant.

- Transfer the roasted peanuts to a bowl and add vinegar, chili powder, and lime zest.
- Toss to coat well and serve.

Nutrition:
Calories: 447
Fat: 39.5g
Carbs: 12.3 g
Protein: 18.9 g
Sodium: 160 mg
Potassium: 200mg
Phosphorus: 0mg

Popcorn with Sugar and Spice

Preparation Time: 10 minutes
Cooking Time: 10 minutes
Servings: 2

Ingredients:
- 8 cups hot popcorn
- 2 tablespoons unsalted butter
- 2 tablespoons sugar
- 1/2 teaspoon cinnamon
- 1/4 teaspoon nutmeg

Directions:
- Popping the corn; put aside.
- Heat the butter, sugar, cinnamon, and nutmeg in the microwave or saucepan over a range fire until the butter is melted, and the sugar dissolved.
- Sprinkle the corn with the spicy butter, mix well.
- Serve immediately for optimal flavor.

Nutrition:
Calories: 120
Fat: 7g
Carbs: 12g
Protein: 2g
Sodium: 2mg
Potassium: 56mg
Phosphorus: 60mg

Eggplant and Chickpea Bites

Preparation Time: 15 minutes
Cooking Time: 50 minutes
Servings: 6

Ingredients:
- 3 large aubergine cut in half (make a few cuts in the flesh with a knife)
- 2 large cloves garlic, peeled and deglazed
- 2 tbsp. coriander powder
- 2 tbsp. cumin seeds
- 400 g canned chickpeas, rinsed and drained
- 2 Tbsp. chickpea flour
- Zest and juice of 1/2 lemon
- 1/2 lemon quartered for serving
- 3 tbsp. tablespoon of polenta

Directions:
- Heat the oven to 200ºC. Spray the eggplant halves generously with oil and place them on the meat side up on a baking sheet.
- Sprinkle with coriander and cumin seeds, and then place the cloves of garlic on the plate.
- Season and roast for 40 minutes until the flesh of eggplant is completely tender. Reserve and let cool a little.
- Scrape the flesh of the eggplant in a bowl with a spatula and throw the skins in the compost. Thoroughly scrape and make sure to incorporate spices and crushed roasted garlic.
- Add chickpeas, chickpea flour, zest, and lemon juice. Crush roughly and mix well.
- Check to season. Do not worry if the mixture seems a bit soft - it will firm up in the fridge.
- Form about twenty pellets and place them on a baking sheet covered with parchment paper. Refrigerate for at least 30 minutes.
- Preheat oven to 180ºC. Remove the meatballs from the fridge and coat them by rolling them in the polenta.
- Place them back on the baking sheet and spray a little oil on each. Roast for 20 minutes until golden and crisp.
- Serve with lemon wedges. You can also serve these dumplings with a spicy yogurt dip.

Nutrition:
Calories: 72
Fat: 1g
Carbs: 18g
Protein: 3g
Sodium: 63mg
Potassium: 162mg
Phosphorus: 36mg

Baba Ghanouj

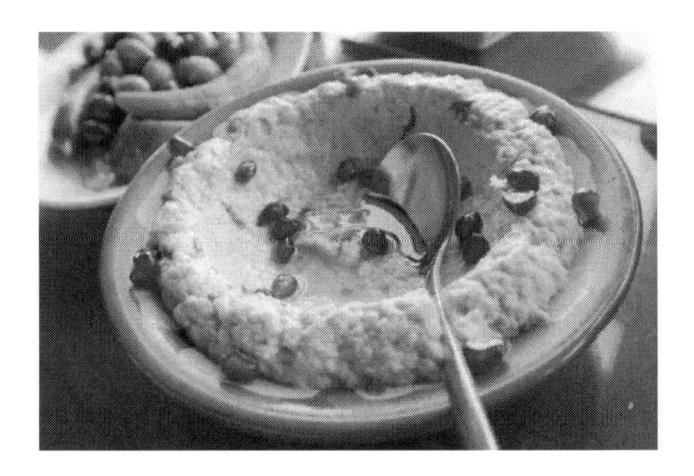

Preparation Time: 10 minutes
Cooking Time: 1 hour and 20 minutes
Servings: 1

Ingredients:
- large aubergine, cut in half lengthwise
- head of garlic, unpeeled
- 30 ml (2 tablespoons) of olive oil
- Lemon juice to taste

Directions:
- Preheat the oven to 350 degrees F.
- Place the eggplant on the plate, skin side up. Roast until the meat is very tender and detaches easily from the skin, about 1 hour depending on the eggplant's size. Let cool.
- Meanwhile, cut the tip of the garlic cloves. Put garlic cloves in a square aluminum foil. Fold the edges of the sheet and fold together to form a tightly wrapped foil.
- Roast with the eggplant until tender, about 20 minutes. Let cool. Purée the pods with a garlic press.
- With a spoon, scoop out the eggplant's flesh and place it in the bowl of a food processor. Add the garlic puree, the oil, and the lemon juice. Stir until purée is smooth and pepper.
- Serve with mini pita bread.

Nutrition:
Calories: 110
Fat: 12g
Carbs: 5g
Protein: 1g
Sodium: 180mg
Potassium: 207mg
Phosphorus: 81mg

Baked Pita Fries

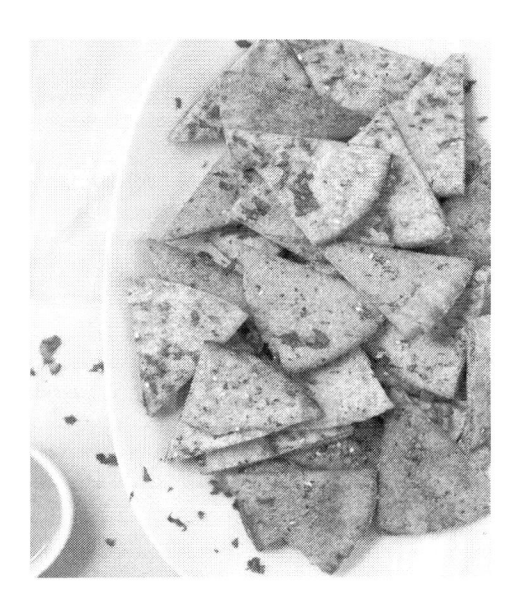

Preparation Time: 5 minutes
Cooking Time: 15 minutes
Servings: 6

Ingredients:
- 3 pita loaves (6 inches)
- 3 tablespoons olive oil
- Chili powder

Directions:
- Separate each bread in half with scissors to obtain 6 round pieces.
- Cut each piece into eight points. Brush each with olive oil and sprinkle with chili powder.
- Bake at 350 degrees F for about 15 minutes until crisp.

Nutrition:
Calories: 120
Fat: 2.5g
Carbs: 22g
Protein: 3g
Sodium: 70mg
Potassium: 0mg
Phosphorus: 0mg

Herbal Cream Cheese Tartines

Preparation Time: 15 minutes
Cooking Time: 15 minutes
Servings: 2

Ingredients:
- clove garlic, halved
- cup cream cheese spread
- ¼ cup chopped herbs such as chives, dill, parsley, tarragon, or thyme
- tbsp. minced French shallot or onion
- ½ tsp. black pepper
- tbsp. tablespoons water

Directions:
- In a medium-sized bowl, combine the cream cheese, herbs, shallot, pepper, and water with a hand blender.
- Serve the cream cheese with the rusks.

Nutrition:
Calories: 476
Fat: 9g
Carbs: 75g
Protein: 23g
Sodium: 885mg
Potassium: 312mg
Phosphorus: 165mg

Mixes of Snacks

Preparation Time: 15 minutes
Cooking Time: 1 hour
Servings: 1

Ingredients:
- 6 c. margarine
- 2 tbsp. Worcestershire sauce
- 1 ½ tbsp. spice salt
- ¾ c. garlic powder
- ½ tsp. onion powder

- 3 cups Cheerios
- 3 cups corn flakes
- 1 cup pretzel
- 1 cup broken bagel chip into 1-inch pieces

Directions:
- Preheat the oven to 250F (120C)
- Melt the margarine in a large roasting pan. Stir in the seasoning. Gradually add the ingredients remaining by mixing so that the coating is uniform.
- Cook 1 hour, stirring every 15 minutes.
- Spread on paper towels to let cool. Store in a tightly closed container.

Nutrition:
Calories: 150
Fat: 6g
Carbs: 20g
Protein: 3g
Sodium: 300mg
Potassium: 93mg
Phosphorus: 70mg

Spicy Crab Dip

Preparation Time: 10 minutes
Cooking Time: 20 minutes
Servings: 1

Ingredients:
- can of 8 oz. softened cream cheese
- tbsp. finely chopped onions
- tbsp. lemon juice
- tbsp. Worcestershire sauce
- 1/8 tsp. black pepper Cayenne pepper to taste
- tbsp. to s. of milk or non-fortified rice drink
- can of 6 oz. of crabmeat

Directions:
- Preheat the oven to 375 degrees F.
- Pour the cheese cream into a bowl. Add the onions, lemon juice, Worcestershire sauce, black pepper, and cayenne pepper. Mix well. Stir in the milk/rice drink.
- Add the crabmeat and mix until you obtain a homogeneous mixture.

- Pour the mixture into a baking dish. Cook without covering for 15 minutes or until bubbles appear. Serve hot with triangle cut pita bread.
- Microwave until bubbles appear, about 4 minutes, stirring every 1 to 2 minutes.

Nutrition:
Calories: 42
Fat: 0.5g
Carbs: 2g
Protein: 7g
Sodium: 167mg
Potassium: 130mg
Phosphorus: 139mg

Baked Apples with Cherries and Walnuts

Preparation Time: 10 minutes
Cooking Time: 35 to 40 minutes
Servings: 6

Ingredients:
- 1/3 cup dried cherries, coarsely chopped
- 3 tablespoons chopped walnuts
- 1 tablespoon ground flaxseed meal
- 1 tablespoon firmly packed brown sugar
- 1 teaspoon ground cinnamon
- 1/8 teaspoon nutmeg
- 6 Golden Delicious apples, about 2 pounds total weight, washed and unpeeled
- 1/2 cup 100 percent apple juice
- 1/4 cup water
- 2 tablespoons dark honey
- 2 teaspoons extra-virgin olive oil

Directions:
- Preheat the oven to 350°F.
- In a small bowl, toss together the cherries, walnuts, flaxseed meal, brown sugar, cinnamon, and nutmeg until all the ingredients are evenly distributed. Set aside.
- Working from the stem end, core each apple, stopping ¾ of an inch from the bottom.
- Gently press the cherries into each apple cavity. Arrange the apples upright in a heavy ovenproof skillet or baking dish just large enough to hold them.
- Pour the apple juice and water into the pan.

- Drizzle the honey and oil evenly over the apples, and cover the pan snugly with aluminum foil. Bake until the apples are tender when pierced with a knife, 35 to 40 minutes.
- Transfer the apples to individual plates and drizzle with the pan juices. Serve warm.

NUTRITION:
Calories: 162;
Total Fat 5g;
Saturated Fat: 1g;
Cholesterol: 0mg;
Sodium: 4mg;
Potassium: 148mg;
Total Carbohydrate: 30g;
Fiber: 4g;
Protein: 1g

Easy Peach Crumble

Preparation Time: 10 minutes
Cooking Time: 30 minutes
Servings: 8

Ingredients:
- 8 ripe peaches, peeled, pitted and sliced
- 3 tablespoons freshly squeezed lemon juice
- 1/2 teaspoon ground cinnamon
- 1/4 teaspoon ground nutmeg
- 1/2 cup oat flour
- 1/4 cup packed dark brown sugar
- 2 tablespoons margarine, cut into thin slices
- 1/4 cup quick-cooking oats

Directions:
- Preheat the oven to 375°F. Lightly coat a 9-inch pie pan with cooking spray. Arrange peach slices in the prepared pie plate and sprinkle with the lemon juice, cinnamon, and nutmeg.
- In a small bowl, whisk together the flour and brown sugar. With your fingers, crumble the margarine into the flour-sugar mixture. Add the uncooked oats and stir to mix. Sprinkle the flour mixture over the peaches.
- Bake until the peaches are soft and the topping is browned, about 30 minutes.
- Cut into 8 even slices and serve warm.

NUTRITION: Calories: 130; Total Fat 4g; Saturated Fat: 0g; Cholesterol: 0mg; Sodium: 42mg; Potassium: 255mg; Total Carbohydrate: 28g; Fiber: 3g; Protein: 2g

CHAPTER 9:
40 RECIPES FOR THOSE WHO HAVE DIALYSIS: BREAKFAST

Breakfast Salad from Grains and Fruits

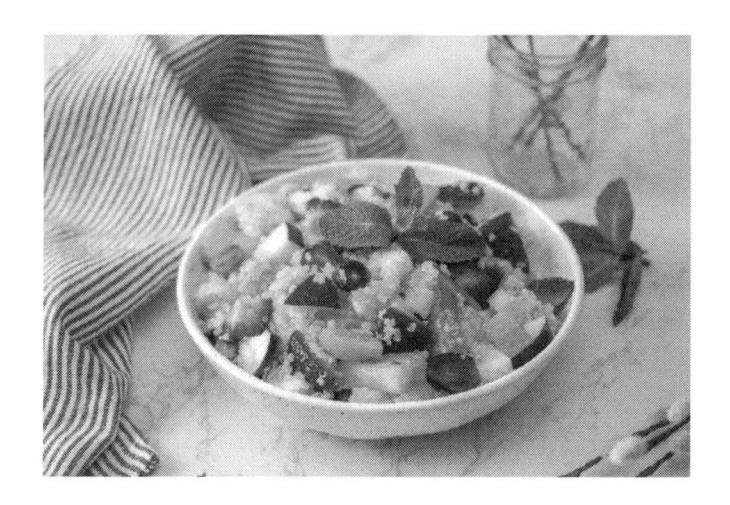

Preparation Time: 5 minutes
Cooking Time: 15 minutes
Servings: 6

Ingredients:
- 8-oz low fat vanilla yogurt
- orange
- Red delicious apple
- Granny Smith apple
- ¾ cup bulgur
- ¼ teaspoon salt
- cups water

Direction:
- On high fire, place a large pot and bring water to a boil.
- Add bulgur and rice. Lower fire to a simmer and cooks for ten minutes while covered.
- Turn off fire, set aside for 2 minutes while covered.
- In baking sheet, transfer and evenly spread grains to cool.
- Meanwhile, peel oranges and cut into sections. Chop and core apples.
- Once grains are cool, transfer to a large serving bowl along with fruits.

- Add yogurt and mix well to coat.
- Serve and enjoy.

Nutrition:
Calories: 187; Carbs: g;
Protein: g;
Fats: g;
Phosphorus: mg;
Potassium: mg;
Sodium: 117mg

French toast with Applesauce

Preparation Time: 5 minutes
Cooking Time: 15 minutes
Servings: 6

Ingredients:
- ¼ cup unsweetened applesauce
- ½ cup milk
- teaspoon ground cinnamon
- eggs
- tablespoon white sugar

Directions:
- Mix well applesauce, sugar, cinnamon, milk and eggs in a mixing bowl.
- Soak the bread, one by one into applesauce mixture until wet.
- On medium fire, heat a nonstick skillet greased with cooking spray.
- Add soaked bread one at a time and cook for 2-3 minutes per side or until lightly browned.
- Serve and enjoy.

Nutrition:
Calories: 57;
Carbs: 6g;
Protein: 4g;
Fats: 4g;
Phosphorus: 69mg;
Potassium: 88mg;
Sodium: 43mg

Bagels Made Healthy

Preparation Time: 5 minutes
Cooking Time: 25 minutes
Servings: 8

Ingredients:
- 2 teaspoon yeast
- ½ tablespoon olive oil
- ¼ cups bread flour
- cups whole wheat flour
- tablespoon vinegar
- tablespoon honey
- ½ cups warm water

Directions:
- In a bread machine, mix all ingredients, and then process on dough cycle.
- Once done or end of cycle, create 8 pieces shaped like a flattened ball.
- In the centre of each ball, make a hole using your thumb then create a donut shape.
- In a greased baking sheet, place donut-shaped dough then covers and let it rise about ½ hour.
- Prepare about 2 inches of water to boil in a large pan.
- In a boiling water, drop one at a time the bagels and boil for 1 minute, then turn them once.
- Remove them and return them to baking sheet and bake at 350oF (175oC) for about 20 to 25 minutes until golden brown.

Nutrition:
Calories: 221;
Carbs: 42g;
Protein: 7g;
Fats: g;
Phosphorus: 130mg;
Potassium: 166mg;
Sodium: 47mg

Cornbread with Southern Twist

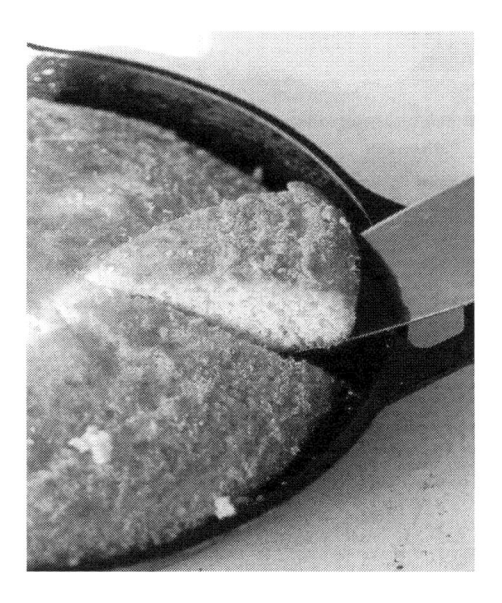

Preparation Time: 15 minutes
Cooking Time: 60 minutes
Servings: 8

Ingredients:
- 2 tablespoons shortening
- 1 ¼ cups skim milk
- ¼ cup egg substitute
- 4 tablespoons sodium free baking powder
- ½ cup flour
- 1 ½ cups cornmeal

Directions:
- Prepare 8 x 8-inch baking dish or a black iron skillet then add shortening.
- Put the baking dish or skillet inside the oven on 425oF, once the shortening has melted that means the pan is hot already.
- In a bowl, add milk and egg then mix well.
- Take out the skillet and add the melted shortening into the batter and stir well.
- Pour all mixed ingredients into skillet.
- For 15 to 20 minutes, cook in the oven until golden brown.

Nutrition:
Calories: 166;
Carbs: 35g;
Protein: 5g;
Fats: 1g;

Phosphorus: 79mg;
Potassium: 122mg;
Sodium: 34mg

Grandma's Pancake Special

Preparation Time: 5 minutes
Cooking Time: 15 minutes
Servings: 3

Ingredients:
- tablespoon oil
- cup milk
- egg
- teaspoons sodium free baking powder
- tablespoons sugar
- ¼ cups flour

Directions:
- Mix together all the dry ingredients such as the flour, sugar and baking powder.
- Combine oil, milk and egg in another bowl. Once done, add them all to the flour mixture.
- Make sure that as your stir the mixture, blend them together until slightly lumpy.
- In a hot greased griddle, pour-in at least ¼ cup of the batter to make each pancake.
- To cook, ensure that the bottom is a bit brown, then turn and cook the other side, as well.

Nutrition:
Calories: 167;
Carbs: 50g;
Protein: 11g;
Fats: 11g;
Phosphorus: 176mg;
Potassium: 215mg;
Sodium: 70mg

Pasta with Indian Lentils

Preparation Time: 5 minutes
Cooking Time: 0 minutes
Servings: 6

Ingredients:
- ¼-½ cup fresh cilantro (chopped)
- cups water
- small dry red peppers (whole)
- teaspoon turmeric
- teaspoon ground cumin
- 2-3 cloves garlic (minced)
- can (15 ounces) cubed Red bell peppers (with juice)
- large onion (chopped)
- ½ cup dry lentils (rinsed)
- ½ cup orzo or tiny pasta

Directions:
- In a skillet, combine all ingredients except for the cilantro then boil on medium-high heat.
- Ensure to cover and slightly reduce heat to medium-low and simmer until pasta is tender for about 35 minutes.
- Afterwards, take out the chili peppers then add cilantro and top it with low-fat sour cream.

Nutrition:
Calories: 175;
Carbs: 40g;
Protein: 3g;
Fats: 2g;
Phosphorus: 139mg;
Potassium: 513mg;
Sodium: 61mg

Shrimp Bruschetta

Preparation Time: 15 minutes
Cooking Time: 10 minutes
Servings: 4

Ingredients:
- 13 oz. shrimps, peeled
- 1 tablespoon tomato sauce

- ½ teaspoon Splenda
- ¼ teaspoon garlic powder
- 1 teaspoon fresh parsley, chopped
- ½ teaspoon olive oil
- 1 teaspoon lemon juice
- 4 whole-grain bread slices
- 1 cup water, for cooking

Directions:
- In the saucepan, pour water and bring it to boil.
- Add shrimps and boil them over the high heat for 5 minutes.
- After this, drain shrimps and chill them to the room temperature.
- Mix up together shrimps with Splenda, garlic powder, tomato sauce, and fresh parsley.
- Add lemon juice and stir gently.
- Preheat the oven to 360f.
- Coat the slice of bread with olive oil and bake for 3 minutes.
- Then place the shrimp mixture on the bread. Bruschetta is cooked.

Nutrition:
Calories 199,
Fat 3.7,
Fiber 2.1,
Carbs 15.3,
Protein 24.1
Calcium 79mg,
Phosphorous 316mg,
Potassium 227mg
Sodium: 121 mg

Strawberry Muesli

Preparation Time: 10 minutes
Cooking Time: 30 minutes
Servings: 4

Ingredients:
- 2 cups Greek yogurt
- ½ cup strawberries, sliced
- ½ cup Muesli
- 4 teaspoon maple syrup
- ¾ teaspoon ground cinnamon

Directions:
- Put Greek yogurt in the food processor.
- Add 1 cup of strawberries, maple syrup, and ground cinnamon.
- Blend the ingredients until you get smooth mass.
- Transfer the yogurt mass in the serving bowls.
- Add Muesli and stir well.
- Leave the meal for 30 minutes in the fridge.
- After this, decorate it with remaining sliced strawberries.

Nutrition:
Calories 149,
Fat 2.6,
Fiber 3.6,
Carbs 21.6,
Protein 12
Calcium 69mg,
Phosphorous 216mg,
Potassium 227mg
Sodium: 151 mg

Yogurt Bulgur

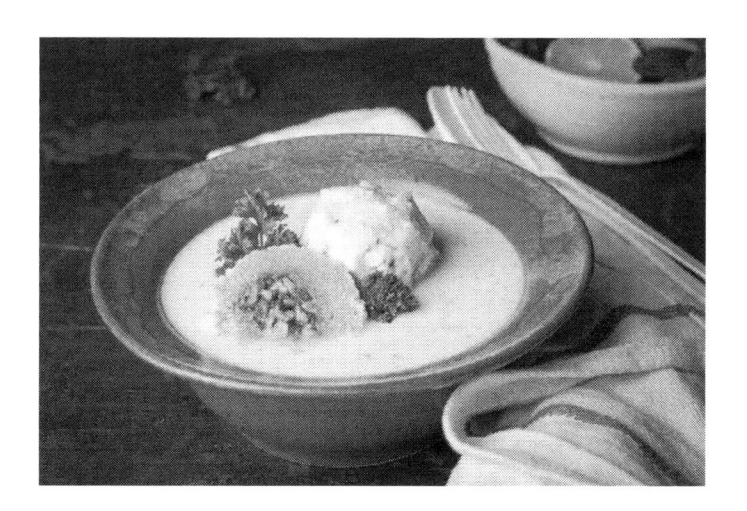

Preparation Time: 10 minutes
Cooking Time: 15 minutes
Servings: 3

Ingredients:
- 1 cup bulgur
- 2 cups Greek yogurt

- 1 ½ cup water
- ½ teaspoon salt
- 1 teaspoon olive oil

Directions:
- Pour olive oil in the saucepan and add bulgur.
- Roast it over the medium heat for 2-3 minutes. Stir it from time to time.
- After this, add salt and water.
- Close the lid and cook bulgur for 15 minutes over the medium heat.
- Then chill the cooked bulgur well and combine it with Greek yogurt. Stir it carefully.
- Transfer the cooked meal into the serving plates. The yogurt bulgur tastes the best when it is cold.

Nutrition:
Calories 274,
Fat 4.9,
Fiber 8.5,
Carbs 40.8,
Protein 19.2
Calcium 39mg,
Phosphorous 216mg,
Potassium 237mg
Sodium: 131 mg

Mozzarella Cheese Omelet

Preparation Time: 10 minutes
Cooking Time: 5 minutes
Servings: 1

Ingredients:
- 4 eggs, beaten
- 1/4 cup mozzarella cheese, shredded
- 4 tomato slices
- 1/4 tsp. Italian seasoning
- 1/4 tsp. dried oregano
- Pepper
- Salt

Directions:
- In a small bowl, whisk eggs with salt.
- Spray pan with cooking spray and heat over medium heat.
- Pour egg mixture into the pan and cook over medium heat.

- Once eggs are set then sprinkle oregano and Italian seasoning on top.
- Arrange tomato slices on top of the omelet and sprinkle with shredded cheese.
- Cook omelet for 1 minute.
- Serve and enjoy.

Nutrition:
Calories 285
 Fat 19g
Carbohydrates 4g
Sugar 3g
Protein 25g
Cholesterol 655 mg

CHAPTER 10:

LUNCH

Couscous and Sherry Vinaigrette

Preparation Time: 10 minutes
Cooking Time: 30 minutes
Servings: 6

Ingredients:

For Sherry Vinaigrette: (makes 2/3 cup)
- 2 tablespoons sherry vinegar
- ¼ cup lemon juice
- clove garlic, pressed
- 1/3 cup olive oil

For Roasted Carrots, Cranberries and Couscous:
- medium onion, sliced
- large carrots, sliced
- tablespoons extra-virgin olive oil
- 2 cups pearl couscous
- 2 ½ to 3 cups no sodium vegetable broth
- ½ cup dried cranberries
- ¼ cup Sherry vinaigrette

Directions:

For Sherry Vinaigrette:
- Beat the vinegar with garlic and lemon juice.
- Slowly whisk in olive oil.
- Store refrigerated in a glass jar.

For Carrots, Cranberries and Couscous:
- Preheat oven to 400°F.
- Spray a baking dish with cooking spray (olive oil) and place the carrots and onions on it.
- Roast the vegetables in oven for about 20 minutes until starting to brown. Stir halfway cooking.
- Heat the couscous in a pan over medium-high heat.
- Toast the couscous until light brown (about 10 minutes). Stir well.
- Check the package instructions for the amount of liquid needed for couscous.

- Bring to a boil the added vegetable stock. Cover and reduce for about 10 minutes. The vegetable stock has to be absorbed.
- In a mixing bowl, incorporate the couscous with the onions, carrots, cranberries, and sherry vinaigrette.
- Serve and enjoy!

Nutrition: Calories 365 Fat 11 g Cholesterol 0 mg Carbohydrate 58 g Sugar 11 g Fiber 4 g Protein 9 g Sodium 95 mg Calcium 41 mg Phosphorus 119 mg Potassium 264 mg

Persian Chicken

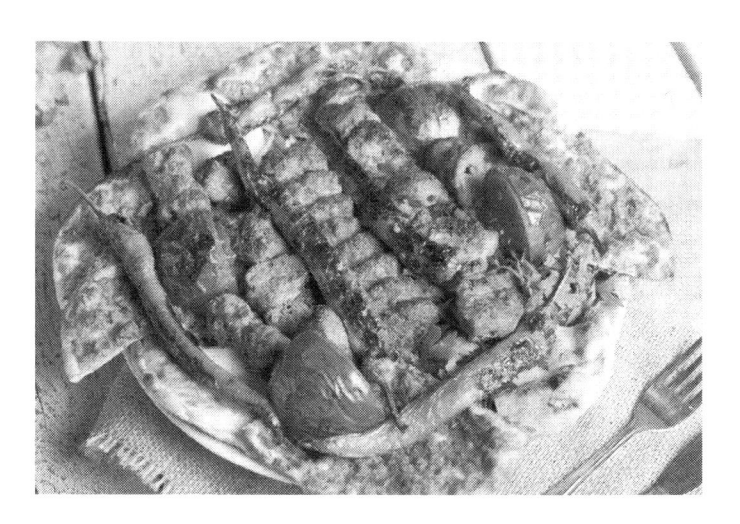

Preparation Time: 10 minutes,
Cooking Time: 20 minutes
Servings: 6

Ingredients:
- ½ small sweet onion,
- ¼ cup freshly squeezed lemon juice
- 1 tablespoon dried oregano
- 1/2 tablespoon of sweet paprika,
- ½ tablespoon of ground cumin
- ½ cup olive oil
- 6 boneless, skinless chicken thighs

Directions:
- Put the vegetables in a blender. Mix it well.
- Put the olive while the motor is running.

- In a sealable bag for the freezer, place the chicken thighs and put the mixture in the sealable bag.
- Refrigerate it for 2 hours, while turning it two times.
- Remove the marinade thighs and discard the additional marinade. Preheat to medium the barbecue. Grill the chicken, turning once or until the internal

Nutrition:
Fat: 21 g;
Carbohydrates: 3 g;
Potassium: 220 mg;
Sodium: 86 mg;
Protein: 22 g

Ratatouille

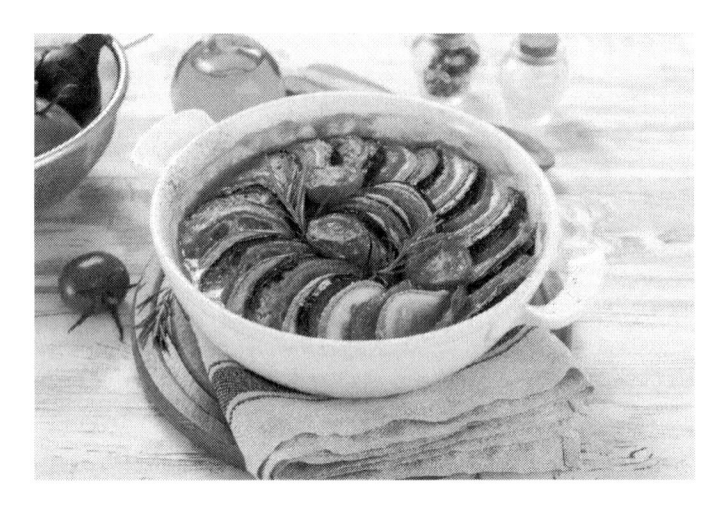

Preparation Time: 5 minutes
Cooking Time: 15 minutes
Servings: 4

Ingredients:
- 1 cup Water
- 3 tbsp. oil
- 2 Zucchinis, sliced in rings
- 2 Eggplants, sliced in rings
- 1 medium Red Onion, sliced in thin rings
- 3 cloves Garlic, minced
- 2 sprigs Fresh Thyme
- Salt to taste

- Black Pepper to taste
- 4 tsp Plain Vinegar

Directions:
- Place all veggies in a bowl, sprinkle with salt and pepper; toss. Line foil in a spring form tin and arrange 1 slice each of the vegetables in, one after the other in a tight circular arrangement.
- Fill the entire tin. Sprinkle the garlic over, some more black pepper and salt, and arrange the thyme sprigs on top. Drizzle olive oil and vinegar over the veggies.
- Place a trivet to fit in the Instant Pot, pour the water in and place the veggies on the trivet. Seal the lid, secure the pressure valve and select Manual mode on High Pressure for 6 minutes. Once ready, quickly release the pressure. Carefully remove the tin and serve ratatouille.

Nutrition:
Calories 152,
Protein 2g,
Net Carbs 4g,
Fat 12g

Jicama Noodles

Preparation Time: 15 minutes
Cooking Time: 7 minutes
Servings: 6

Ingredients:
- 1-pound jicama, peeled
- 2 tablespoons butter
- teaspoon chili flakes
- teaspoon salt
- ¾ cup of water

Directions:
- Spiralize jicama with the help of spiralizer and place in jicama spirals in the saucepan.
- Add butter, chili flakes, and salt.
- Then add water and preheat the ingredients until the butter is melted.
- Mix up it well.
- Close the lid and cook noodles for 4 minutes over the medium heat.
- Stir the jicama noodles well before transferring them in the serving plates.

Nutrition:
Calories 63,
Fat 3.9,

Fiber 3.7,
Carbs 6.7,
Protein 0.6

Crack Slaw

Preparation Time: 15 minutes
Cooking Time: 10 minutes
Servings: 6

Ingredients:
- 1 cup cauliflower rice
- 1 tablespoon sriracha
- 1 teaspoon tahini paste
- 1 teaspoon sesame seeds
- 1 tablespoon lemon juice
- 1 teaspoon olive oil
- 1 teaspoon butter
- ½ teaspoon salt
- 2 cups coleslaw

Directions:
- Toss the butter in the skillet and melt it.
- Add cauliflower rice and sprinkle it with sriracha and tahini paste.
- Mix up the vegetables and cook them for 10 minutes over the medium heat. Stir them from time to time.
- When the cauliflower is cooked, transfer it into the big plate.
- Add coleslaw and stir gently.
- Then sprinkle the salad with sesame seeds, lemon juice, olive oil, and salt.
- Mix up well.

Nutrition: Calories 76, Fat 5.8, Fiber 0.6, Carbs 6, Protein 1.1

Vegan Chili

Preparation Time: 10 minutes
Cooking Time: 20 minutes
Servings: 4

Ingredients:
- 1 cup cremini mushrooms, chopped
- 1 zucchini, chopped
- 1 bell pepper, diced
- 1/3 cup crushed Red bell peppers
- 1 oz. celery stalk, chopped
- 1 teaspoon chili powder
- 1 teaspoon salt
- ½ teaspoon chili flakes
- ½ cup of water
- 1 tablespoon olive oil
- ½ teaspoon diced garlic
- ½ teaspoon ground black pepper
- 1 teaspoon of cocoa powder
- 2 oz. Cheddar cheese, grated

Directions:
- Pour olive oil in the pan and preheat it.
- Add chopped mushrooms and roast them for 5 minutes. Stir them from time to time.
- After this, add chopped zucchini and bell pepper.

- Sprinkle the vegetables with the chili powder, salt, chili flakes, diced garlic, and ground black pepper.
- Stir the vegetables and cook them for 5 minutes more.
- After this, add crushed Red bell peppers. Mix up well.
- Bring the mixture to boil and add water and cocoa powder.
- Then add celery stalk.
- Mix up the chili well and close the lid.
- Cook the chili for 10 minutes over the medium-low heat.
- Then transfer the cooked vegan chili in the bowls and top with the grated cheese.

Nutrition:
Calories 123,
Fat 8.6,
Fiber 2.3,
Carbs 7.6,
Protein 5.6

Chow Mein

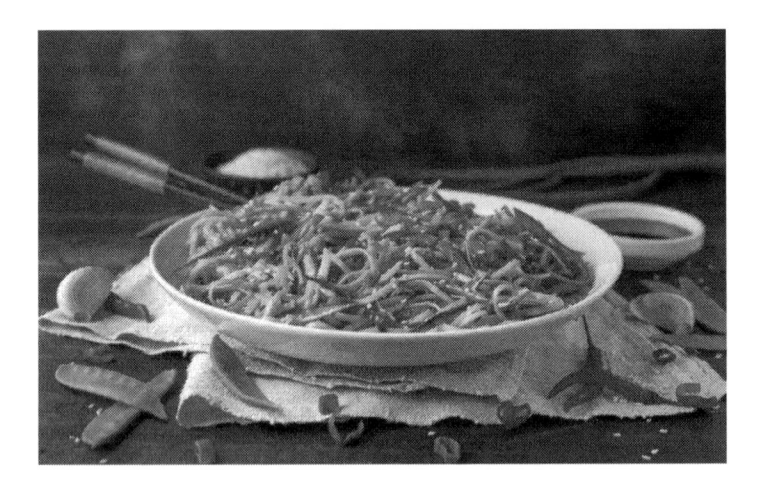

Preparation Time: 10 minutes
Cooking Time: 10 minutes
Servings: 6

Ingredients:
- 7 oz. kelp noodles
- 5 oz. broccoli florets
- 1 tablespoon tahini sauce
- ¼ teaspoon minced ginger
- 1 teaspoon Sriracha
- ½ teaspoon garlic powder
- 1 cup of water

Directions:
- Boil water in a sauce pan.
- Add broccoli and boil for 4 minutes over the high heat.
- Then drain water into the bowl and chill it tills the room temperature.
- Soak the kelp noodles in the "broccoli water".
- Meanwhile, place tahini sauce, sriracha, minced ginger, and garlic in the saucepan.
- Bring the mixture to boil. Add oil if needed.
- Then add broccoli and soaked noodles.
- Add 3 tablespoons of "broccoli water".
- Mix up the noodles and bring to boil.
- Switch off the heat and transfer chow Mein in the serving bowls.

Nutrition:
Calories 18,
Fat 0.8,

Fiber 0.7,
Carbs 2.8,
Protein 0.9

Mushroom Tacos

Preparation Time: 10 minutes
Cooking Time: 15 minutes
Servings: 6

Ingredients:
- 6 collard greens leave
- 2 cups mushrooms, chopped
- 1 white onion, diced
- 1 tablespoon Taco seasoning
- 1 tablespoon coconut oil
- ½ teaspoon salt
- ¼ cup fresh parsley
- 1 tablespoon mayonnaise

Directions:
- Put the coconut oil in the skillet and melt it.
- Add chopped mushrooms and diced onion. Mix up the ingredients.
- Close the lid and cook them for 10 minutes.
- After this, sprinkle the vegetables with Taco seasoning, salt, and add fresh parsley.
- Mix up the mixture and cook for 5 minutes more.
- Then add mayonnaise and stir well.
- Chill the mushroom mixture little.
- Fill the collard green leaves with the mushroom mixture and fold up them.

Nutrition: Calories 52, Fat 3.3, Fiber 1.2, Carbs 5.1, Protein 1.4

Lime Green lettuce and Chickpeas Salad

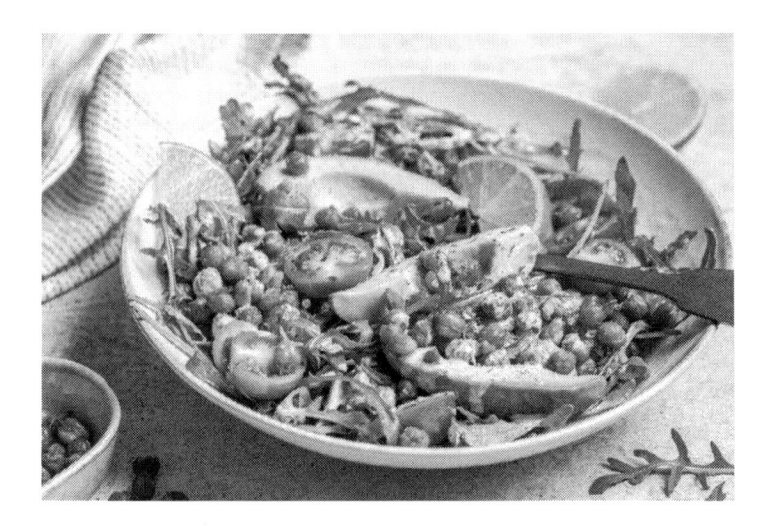

Preparation Time: 10 minutes
Cooking Time: 0 minutes
Servings: 4

Ingredients:
- 16 ounces canned chickpeas, drained and rinsed
- 2 cups baby green lettuce leaves
- ½ tablespoon lime juice
- 2 tablespoons olive oil
- 1 teaspoon cumin, ground
- Sea salt and black pepper
- ½ teaspoon chili flakes

Directions:
- In a bowl, mix the chickpeas with the green lettuce and the rest of the ingredients, toss and serve cold.

Nutrition:
Calories 240,
Fat 8.2,
Fiber 5.3,
Carbs 11.6,
Protein 12

Fried Rice with Kale

Preparation Time: 10 minutes
Cooking Time: 12 minutes
Servings: 4

Ingredients:
- 2 tbsp. Extra virgin oil
- 8 oz. Tofu, chopped
- 6 Scallion, white and green parts, thinly sliced
- 2 cups Kale, stemmed and chopped
- 3 cups Cooked white rice
- ¼ cup Stir fry sauce

Directions:
- In a huge skillet on medium-high heat, warm the oil until it shimmers.
- Add the tofu, scallions, and kale. Cook for 5 to 7 minutes, frequently stirring, until the vegetables are soft.
- Add the white rice and stir-fry sauce. Cook for 3 to 5 minutes, occasionally stirring, until heated through.

Nutrition:
Calories: 301
Total Fat: 11g
Total Carbs: 36g
Sugar: 1g
Fiber: 3g
Protein: 16g
Sodium: 2,535mg

Stir-Fried Gingery Veggies

Preparation Time: 10 minutes
Cooking Time: 10 minutes
Servings: 4

Ingredients:
- 1 tablespoon oil
- 3 cloves of garlic, minced
- 1 onion, chopped
- 1 thumb-size ginger, sliced

- 1 tablespoon water
- 1 large carrots, peeled and julienned and seedless
- 1 large green bell pepper, julienned and seedless
- 1 large yellow bell pepper, julienned and seedless
- 1 large red bell pepper, julienned and seedless
- 1 zucchini, julienned
- Salt and pepper to taste

Directions:
- Heat oil in a nonstick saucepan over a high flame and sauté the garlic, onion, and ginger until fragrant.
- Stir in the rest of the ingredients.
- Keep on stirring for at least 5 minutes until vegetables are tender.
- Serve and enjoy.

Nutrition:
Calories 70
Total Fat 4g
Saturated Fat 1g
Total Carbs 9g
Net Carbs 7g
Protein 1g
Sugar: 4g
Fiber 2g
Sodium 173mg
Potassium 163mg

CHAPTER 11:

DINNER

Fish En' Papillote

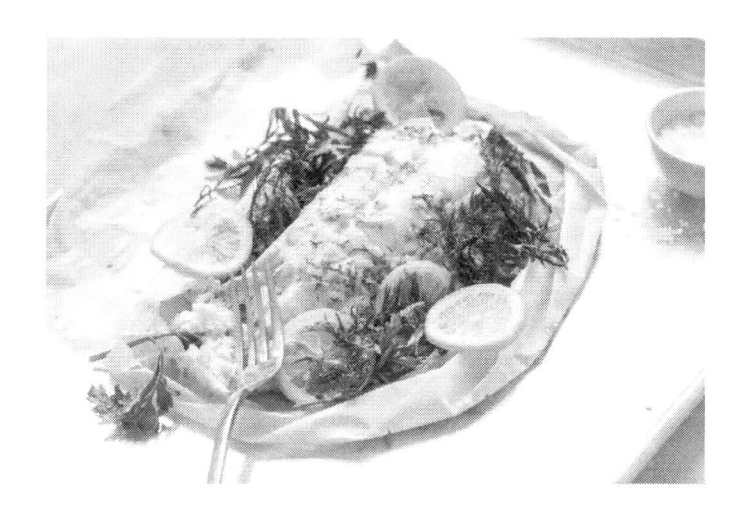

Preparation Time: 15 minutes
Cooking Time: 20 minutes
Servings: 3

Ingredients:
- 10 oz. snapper fillet
- 1 tablespoon fresh dill, chopped
- 1 white onion, peeled, sliced
- ½ teaspoon tarragon
- 1 tablespoon olive oil
- 1 teaspoon salt
- ½ teaspoon hot pepper
- 2 tablespoons sour cream

Directions:
- Make the medium size packets from parchment and arrange them in the baking tray. Cut the snapper fillet into 3 and sprinkle them with salt, tarragon, and hot pepper.
- Put the fish fillets in the parchment packets. Then top the fish with olive oil, sour cream, sliced onion, and fresh dill. Bake the fish for 20 minutes at 355F. Serve.

Nutrition:
Calories 204
Fat 8.2g

Carbs 4.6g
Protein 27.2g
Phosphorus 138.8 mg
Potassium 181.9 mg
Sodium 59.6 mg

Pesto Pasta Salad

Preparation Time: 15 minutes
Cooking Time: 15 minutes
Servings: 4

Ingredients:
- 1 cup fresh basil leaves
- ½ cup packed fresh flat-leaf parsley leaves
- ½ cup arugula, chopped
- 2 tablespoons Parmesan cheese, grated
- ¼ cup extra-virgin olive oil
- 3 tablespoons mayonnaise
- 2 tablespoons water
- 12 ounces whole-wheat rotini pasta
- 1 red bell pepper, chopped
- 1 medium yellow summer squash, sliced
- 1 cup frozen baby peas

Directions:
- Boil water in a large pot.
- Meanwhile, combine the basil, parsley, arugula, cheese, and olive oil in a blender or food processor. Process until the herbs are finely chopped. Add the mayonnaise and water, then process again. Set aside.
- Prepare the pasta to the pot of boiling water; cook according to package directions, about 8 to 9 minutes. Drain well, reserving ¼ cup of the cooking liquid.
- Combine the pesto, pasta, bell pepper, squash, and peas in a large bowl and toss gently, adding enough reserved pasta cooking liquid to make a sauce on the salad. Serve immediately or cover and chill, then serve.
- Store covered in the refrigerator for up to 3 days.

Nutrition:
Calories: 378
Fat: 24g
Carbohydrates: 35g

Protein: 9g
Sodium: 163mg
Potassium: 472mg
Phosphorus: 213mg

Barley Blueberry Salad

Preparation Time: 15 minutes
Cooking Time: 15 minutes
Servings: 4

Ingredients:
- 1 cup quick-cooking barley
- 3 cups low-sodium vegetable broth
- 3 tablespoons extra-virgin olive oil
- 2 tablespoons freshly squeezed lemon juice
- 1 teaspoon yellow mustard
- 1 teaspoon honey
- 2 cups blueberries
- ¼ cup crumbled feta cheese

Directions:
- Combine the barley and vegetable broth in a medium saucepan and bring to a simmer.
- Reduce the heat to low, partially cover the pan, and simmer for 10 to 12 minutes or until the barley is tender.
- Meanwhile, whisk together the olive oil, lemon juice, mustard, and honey in a serving bowl until blended.
- Drain the barley if necessary and add to the bowl; toss to combine.
- Add the blueberries, and feta and toss gently. Serve.

Nutrition:
Calories: 345
Fat 16g
Carbohydrates: 44g
Protein: 7g
Sodium: 259mg
Potassium: 301mg
Phosphorus: 152mg

Pasta with Creamy Broccoli Sauce

Preparation Time: 15 minutes
Cooking Time: 15 minutes
Servings: 4

Ingredients:
- 2 tablespoons olive oil
- 1-pound broccoli florets
- garlic cloves, halved
- cup low-sodium vegetable broth
- ½ pound whole-wheat spaghetti pasta
- ounces cream cheese
- teaspoon dried basil leaves
- ½ cup grated Parmesan cheese

Directions:
- Prepare a large pot of water to a boil.
- Put olive oil in a large skillet. Sauté the broccoli and garlic for 3 minutes.
- Add the broth to the skillet and bring to a simmer. Reduce the heat to low, partially cover the skillet, and simmer until the broccoli is tender about 5 to 6 minutes.
- Cook the pasta according to package directions. Drain when al dente, reserving 1 cup pasta water.
- When the broccoli is tender, add the cream cheese and basil—purée using an immersion blender.
- Put mixture into a food processor, about half at a time, and purée until smooth and transfer the sauce back into the skillet.
- Add the cooked pasta to the broccoli sauce. Toss, adding enough pasta water until the sauce coats the pasta completely. Sprinkle with the Parmesan and serve.

Nutrition:
Calories: 302
Fat 14g
Carbohydrates: 36g
Protein: 11g
Sodium: 260mg
Potassium: 375mg
Phosphorus: 223mg

Asparagus Fried Rice

Preparation Time: 10 minutes
Cooking Time: 10 minutes
Servings: 1

Ingredients:
- 3 large eggs, beaten
- ½ teaspoon ground ginger
- 2 teaspoons low-sodium soy sauce
- 2 tablespoons olive oil
- 1 onion, diced
- 4 garlic cloves, minced
- 1 cup sliced cremini mushrooms
- 1 (10-ounce) package frozen white rice, thawed
- 8 ounces fresh asparagus, about 15 spears, cut into 1-inch pieces
- 1 teaspoon sesame oil

Directions:
- Whisk the eggs, ginger, and soy sauce in a small bowl and set aside.
- Heat the olive oil in a medium skillet or wok over medium heat.
- Add the onion and garlic and sauté for 2 minutes until tender crisp.
- Add the mushrooms and rice; stir-fry for 3 minutes longer.
- Put asparagus and cook for 2 minutes.6.
- Pour in the egg mixture. Stir the eggs until cooked through, 2 to 3 minutes, and stir into the rice mixture.
- Sprinkle the fried rice with the sesame oil and serve.

Nutrition:
Calories: 247
Fat: 13g
Carbohydrates: 25g
Protein: 9g
Sodium: 149mg
Potassium: 367mg
Phosphorus: 206mg

Beef and Chili Stew

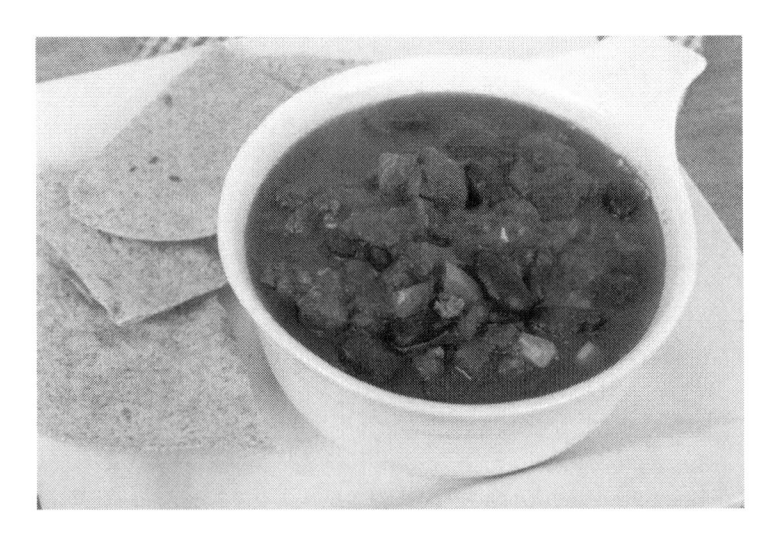

Preparation Time: 15 minutes
Cooking Time: 7 hours
Servings: 6

Ingredients:
- 1/2 medium red onion, sliced thinly
- 1/2 tablespoon vegetable oil
- 10ounce of flat-cut beef brisket, whole
- ½ cup low sodium stock
- ¾ cup of water
- ½ tablespoon honey
- ½ tablespoon chili powder
- ½ teaspoon smoked paprika
- ½ teaspoon dried thyme
- teaspoon black pepper
- tablespoon corn starch

Directions:
- Throw the sliced onion into the slow cooker first. Add a splash of oil to a large hot skillet and briefly seal the beef on all sides.
- Remove the beef, then place it in the slow cooker. Add the stock, water, honey, and spices to the same skillet you cooked the beef meat.
- Allow the juice to simmer until the volume is reduced by about half. Pour the juice over beef in the slow cooker. Cook on low within 7 hours.
- Transfer the beef to your platter, shred it using two forks. Put the rest of the juice into a medium saucepan. Bring it to a simmer.

- Whisk the cornstarch with two tablespoons of water. Add to the juice and cook until slightly thickened.
- For a thicker sauce, simmer and reduce the juice a bit more before adding cornstarch. Put the sauce on the meat and serve.

Nutrition:
Calories: 128
Protein: 13g
Carbohydrates: 6g
Fat: 6g
Sodium: 228mg
Potassium: 202mg
Phosphorus: 119mg

Sticky Pulled Beef Open Sandwiches

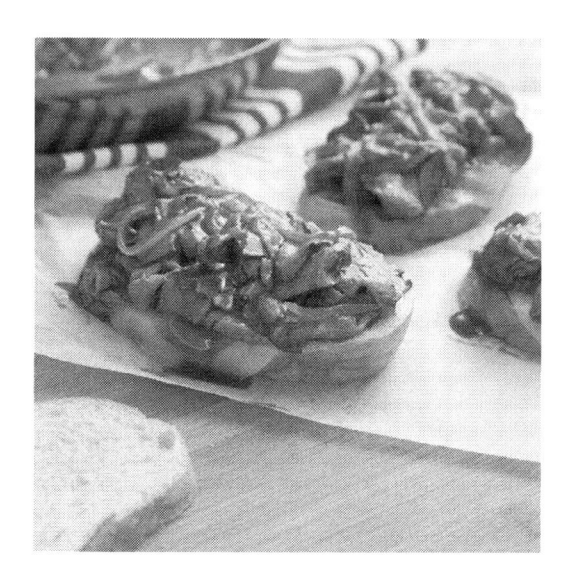

Preparation Time: 15 minutes
Cooking Time: 5 hours
Servings: 5

Ingredients:
- ½ cup of green onion, sliced
- 2 garlic cloves
- 2 tablespoons of fresh parsley
- 2 large carrots
- 7ounce of flat-cut beef brisket, whole

- 1 tablespoon of smoked paprika
- 1 teaspoon dried parsley
- 1 teaspoon of brown sugar
- ½ teaspoon of black pepper
- 2 tablespoon of olive oil
- ¼ cup of red wine
- 8 tablespoon of cider vinegar
- 3 cups of water
- 5 slices white bread
- 1 cup of arugula to garnish

Directions:
- Finely chop the green onion, garlic, and fresh parsley. Grate the carrot. Put the beef in to roast in a slow cooker.
- Add the chopped onion, garlic, and remaining ingredients, leaving the rolls, fresh parsley, and arugula to one side. Stir in the slow cooker to combine.
- Cover and cook on low within 8 1/2 to 10 hours or on high for 4 to 5 hours until tender. Remove the meat from the slow cooker. Shred the meat using two forks.
- Return the meat to the broth to keep it warm until ready to serve. Lightly toast the bread and top with shredded beef, arugula, fresh parsley, and ½ spoon of the broth. Serve.

Nutrition:
Calories: 273
Protein: 15g
Carbohydrates: 20g
Fat: 11g
Sodium: 308mg
Potassium: 399mg
Phosphorus: 159mg

Herby Beef Stroganoff and Fluffy Rice

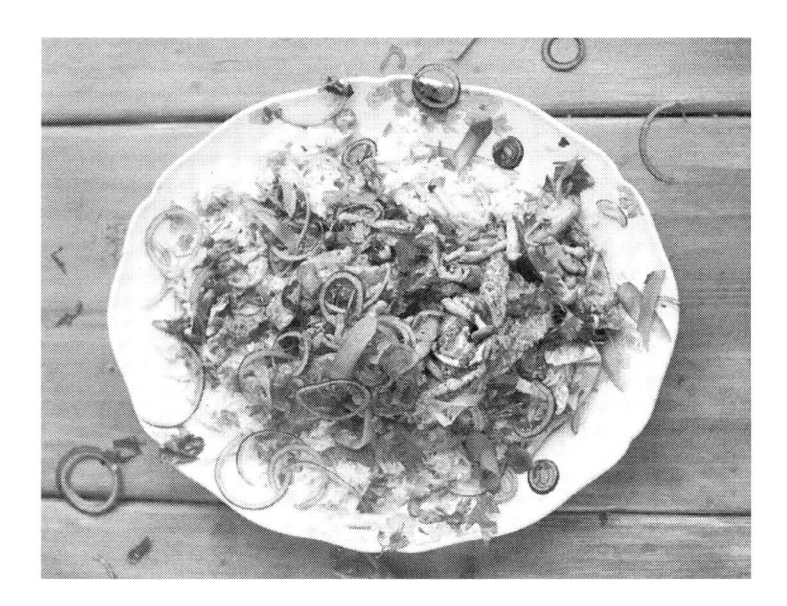

Preparation Time: 15 minutes
Cooking Time: 5 hours
Servings: 6

Ingredients:
- ½ cup onion
- 2 garlic cloves
- 9ounce of flat-cut beef brisket, cut into 1" cubes
- ½ cup of reduced-sodium beef stock
- 1/3 cup red wine
- ½ teaspoon dried oregano
- ¼ teaspoon freshly ground black pepper
- ½ teaspoon dried thyme
- ½ teaspoon of saffron
- ½ cup almond milk (unenriched)
- ¼ cup all-purpose flour
- cup of water
- ½ cups of white rice

Directions:
- Dice the onion, then mince the garlic cloves. Mix the beef, stock, wine, onion, garlic, oregano, pepper, thyme, and saffron in your slow cooker.
- Cover and cook on high within 4-5 hours. Combine the almond milk, flour, and water. Whisk together until smooth.

- Add the flour mixture to the slow cooker. Cook for another 15 to 25 minutes until the stroganoff is thick.
- Cook the rice using the package instructions, leaving out the salt. Drain off the excess water. Serve the stroganoff over the rice.

Nutrition:
Calories: 241
Protein: 15g
Carbohydrates: 29g
Fat: 5g
Sodium: 182mg
Potassium: 206mg
Phosphorus: 151mg

Chunky Beef and Potato Slow Roast

Preparation Time: 15 minutes
Cooking Time: 5-6 hours
Servings: 12

Ingredients:
- 3 cups of peeled potatoes, chunked
- 1 cup of onion
- 2 garlic cloves, chopped
- 1 ¼ pound flat-cut beef brisket, fat trimmed
- 2 cups of water
- 1 teaspoon of chili powder
- 1 tablespoon of dried rosemary

For the sauce:
- tablespoon of freshly grated horseradish
- ½ cup of almond milk (unenriched)
- tablespoon lemon juice (freshly squeezed)
- garlic clove, minced
- A pinch of cayenne pepper

Directions:
- Double boil the potatoes to reduce their potassium content. Chop the onion and the garlic. Place the beef brisket in a slow cooker. Combine water, chopped garlic, chili powder, and rosemary.
- Pour the mixture over the brisket. Cover and cook on high within 4-5 hours until the meat is very tender. Drain the potatoes and add them to the slow cooker.

- Adjust the heat to high and cook covered until the potatoes are tender. Prepare the horseradish sauce by whisking together horseradish, milk, lemon juice, minced garlic, and cayenne pepper.
- Cover and refrigerate. Serve your casserole with a dash of horseradish sauce on the side.

Nutrition:
Calories: 199
Protein: 21g
Carbohydrates: 12g
Fat: 7g
Sodium: 282mg
Potassium: 317
Phosphorus: 191mg

Spiced Lamb Burgers

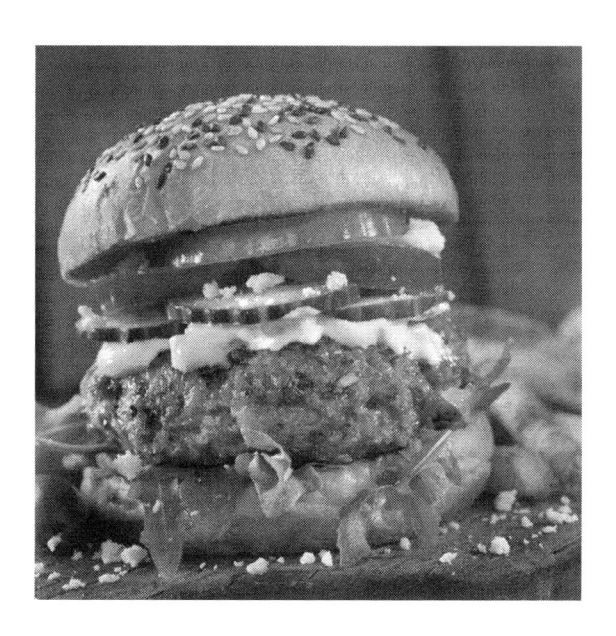

Preparation Time: 10 minutes
Cooking Time: 20 minutes
Servings: 2

Ingredients:
- tablespoon extra-virgin olive oil
- teaspoon cumin
- ½ finely diced red onion
- minced garlic clove
- teaspoon harissa spices

- cup arugula
- juiced lemon
- 6-ounce lean ground lamb
- tablespoon parsley
- ½ cup low-fat plain yogurt

Directions:
- Preheat the broiler on medium to high heat. Mix the ground lamb, red onion, parsley, Harissa spices, and olive oil until combined.
- Shape 1-inch thick patties using wet hands. Add the patties to a baking tray and place under the broiler for 7-8 minutes on each side. Mix the yogurt, lemon juice, and cumin and serve over the lamb burgers with arugula's side salad.

Nutrition:
Calories 306
Fat 20g
Carbs 10g
Phosphorus 269mg
Potassium 492mg
Sodium 86mg
Protein 23g

Pork Loins with Leeks

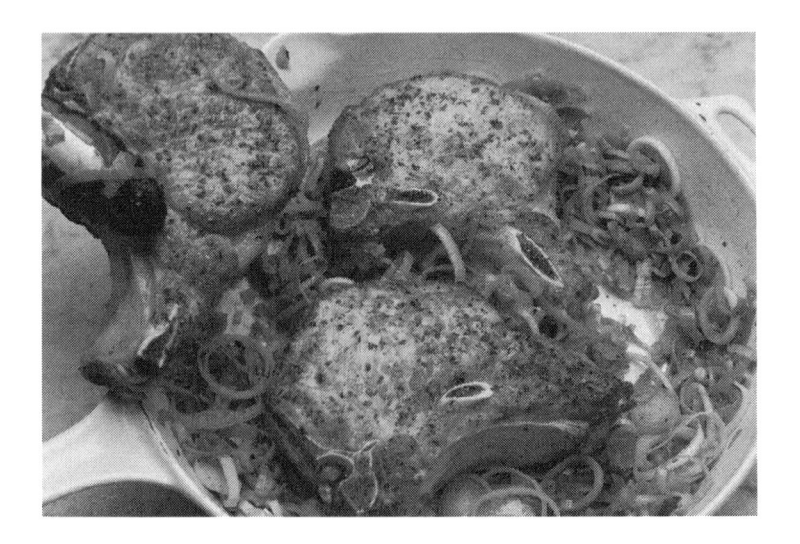

Preparation Time: 10 minutes
Cooking Time: 35 minutes
Servings: 2

Ingredients:
- sliced leek
- tablespoon mustard seeds
- 6-ounce pork tenderloin
- tablespoon cumin seeds
- tablespoon dry mustard
- tablespoon extra-virgin oil

Directions:
- Preheat the broiler to medium-high heat. In a dry skillet, heat mustard and cumin seeds until they start to pop (3-5 minutes). Grind seeds using a pestle and mortar or blender and then mix in the dry mustard.
- Massage the pork on all sides using the mustard blend and add to a baking tray to broil for 25-30 minutes or until cooked through. Turn once halfway through.
- Remove and place to one side, then heat-up the oil in a pan on medium heat and add the leeks for 5-6 minutes or until soft. Serve the pork tenderloin on a bed of leeks and enjoy it!

Nutrition:
Calories 139
Fat 5g
Carbs 2g
Phosphorus 278mg
Potassium 45mg
Sodium 47mg
Protein 18g

The Kale and Green lettuce Soup

Preparation Time: 5 minutes
Cooking Time: 10 minutes
Servings: 4

Ingredients:
- 3 ounces coconut oil
- 8 ounces kale, chopped
- 4 1/3 cups coconut almond milk
- Sunflower seeds and pepper to taste

Directions:
- Take a skillet and place it over medium heat.
- Add kale and sauté for 2-3 minutes

- Add kale to blender.
- Add water, spices, coconut almond milk to blender as well.
- Blend until smooth and pour mix into bowl.
- Serve and enjoy!

Nutrition:
Calories: 124
Fat: 13g
Carbohydrates: 7g
Protein: 4.2g
Phosphorus: 110mg
Potassium: 117mg
Sodium: 105mg

Japanese Onion Soup

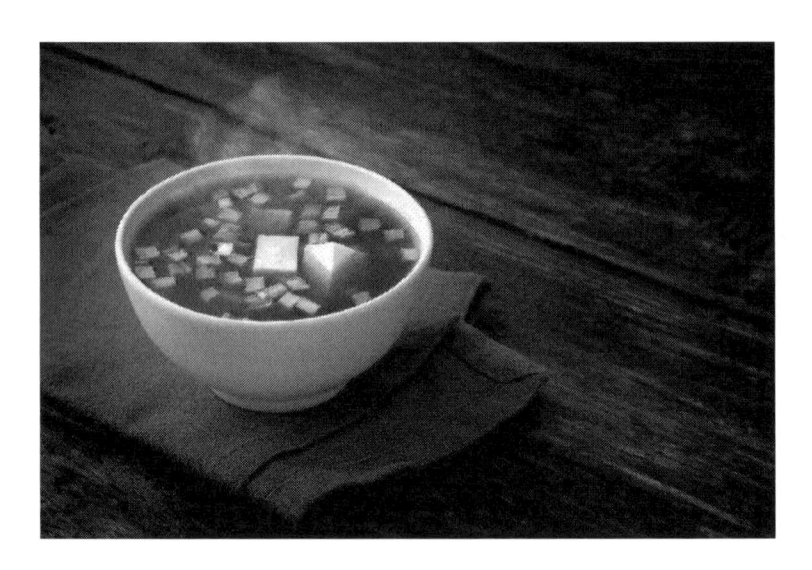

Preparation Time: 15 minutes
Cooking Time: 45 minutes
Servings: 4

Ingredients:
- ½ stalk celery, diced
- 1 small onion, diced
- ½ carrot, diced
- 1 teaspoon fresh ginger root, grated
- ¼ teaspoon fresh garlic, minced
- 2 tablespoons chicken stock

- 3 teaspoons beef bouillon granules
- 1 cup fresh shiitake, mushrooms
- 2 quarts water
- 1 cup baby Portobello mushrooms, sliced
- 1 tablespoon fresh chives

Directions:
- Take a saucepan and place it over high heat, add water, bring to a boil.
- Add beef bouillon, celery, onion, chicken stock, and carrots, half of the mushrooms, ginger, and garlic.
- Put on the lid and reduce heat to medium, cook for 45 minutes.
- Take another saucepan and add another half of mushrooms.
- Once the soup is cooked, strain the soup into the pot with uncooked mushrooms.
- Garnish with chives and enjoy!

Nutrition:
Calories: 25
Fat: 0.2g
Carbohydrates: 5g
Protein: 1.4g
Phosphorus: 210mg
Potassium: 217mg
Sodium: 75mg

Amazing Broccoli and Cauliflower Soup

Preparation Time: 10 minutes
Cooking Time: 8 hours
Servings: 4

Ingredients:

- 3 cups broccoli florets
- 2 cups cauliflower florets
- 2 garlic cloves, minced
- ½ cup shallots, chopped
- 1 carrot, chopped
- 3 ½ cups low sodium veggie stick
- Pinch of pepper

- 1 cup fat-free milk
- 6 ounces low-fat cheddar, shredded
- 1 cup non-fat Greek yogurt

Directions:
- Add broccoli, cauliflower, garlic, shallots, carrot, stock, and pepper to your Slow Cooker.
- Stir well and place lid.
- Cook on LOW for 8 hours.
- Add milk and cheese.
- Use an immersion blender to smooth the soup.
- Add yogurt and blend once more.
- Ladle into bowls and enjoy!

Nutrition:
Calories: 218
Fat: 11g
Carbohydrates: 15g
Protein: 12g
Phosphorus: 206mg
Potassium: 147mg
Sodium: 75mg

CHAPTER 12:

SNACKS

Lemon Thins

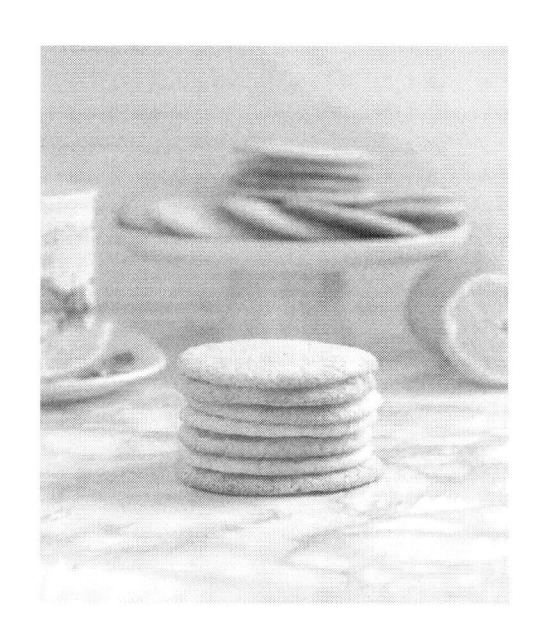

Preparation Time: 15 minutes
Cooking Time: 8 to 10 minutes
Servings: 30 cookies

Ingredients:

- Cooking spray
- 1 1/4 cups whole wheat pastry flour
- 1/3 cup cornstarch
- 1 1/2 teaspoons baking powder
- ¾ cup sugar, divided
- 2 tablespoons butter, softened
- 2 tablespoons extra-virgin olive oil
- 1 large egg white
- 3 teaspoons freshly grated lemon zest
- 1 1/2 teaspoons vanilla extract
- 4 tablespoons freshly squeezed lemon juice

Directions:
- Preheat the oven to 350°F. Coat two baking sheets with cooking spray.
- In a mixing bowl, whisk together the flour, cornstarch, and baking powder.
- In another mixing bowl beat 1/2 cup of the sugar, the butter, and olive oil with an electric mixer on medium speed until fluffy.
- Add the egg white, lemon zest, and vanilla and beat until smooth. Beat in the lemon juice.
- Add the dry ingredients to the wet ingredients and fold in with a rubber spatula just until combined.
- Drop the dough by the teaspoonful, 2 inches apart, onto the prepared baking sheets.
- Place the remaining 1/4 cup sugar in a saucer. Coat the bottom of a wide-bottomed glass with cooking spray and dip it in the sugar. Flatten the dough with the glass bottom into 2 1/2-inch circles, dipping the glass in the sugar each time.
- Bake the cookies until they are just starting to brown around the edges, 8 to 10 minutes. Transfer to a flat surface (not a rack) to crisp.

NUTRITION: (1 cookie) Calories: 40; Total Fat 2g; Saturated Fat: 1g; Cholesterol: 2mg; Sodium: 26mg; Potassium: 3mg; Total Carbohydrate: 5g; Fiber: 1g; Protein: 1g

Snickerdoodle Chickpea Blondies

Servings: 15
Preparation Time: 10 minutes
Cooking Time: 30 to 35 minutes

Ingredients:
- 1 (15-ounce) can chickpeas, drained and rinsed
- 3 tablespoons nut butter of choice
- ¾ teaspoon baking powder
- 2 teaspoons vanilla extract
- 1/8 teaspoon baking soda
- ¾ cup brown sugar
- 1 tablespoon unsweetened applesauce
- 1/4 cup ground flaxseed meal
- 2 1/4 teaspoons cinnamon

Directions:
- Preheat the oven to 350°F. Grease an 8-by-8-inch baking pan.
- Blend all ingredients in a food processor until very smooth. Scoop into the prepared baking pan.

- Bake until the tops are medium golden brown, 30 to 35 minutes. Allow the brownies to cool completely before cutting.

NUTRITION: Calories: 85; Total Fat 2g; Saturated Fat: 0g; Cholesterol: 0mg; Sodium: 7mg; Potassium: 62mg; Total Carbohydrate: 16g; Fiber: 2g; Protein: 3g

Chocolate Chia Seed Pudding

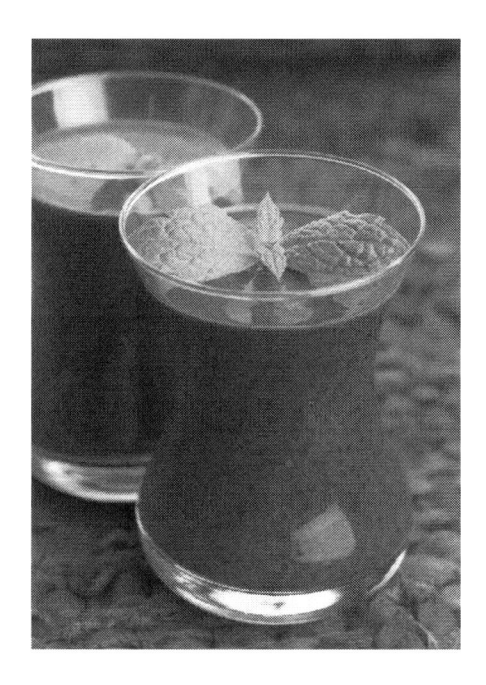

Preparation Time: 15 minutes, plus 3 to 5 hours or overnight to rest
Cooking Time: 0 minutes
Servings: 4

Ingredients:

- 1 1/2 cups unsweetened vanilla almond milk
- 1/4 cup unsweetened cocoa powder
- 1/4 cup maple syrup (or substitute any sweetener)
- 1/2 teaspoon vanilla extract
- 1/3 cup chia seeds
- 1/2 cup strawberries
- 1/4 cup blueberries
- 1/4 cup raspberries

- 2 tablespoons unsweetened coconut flakes
- 1/4 to 1/2 teaspoon ground cinnamon (optional)

Directions:
- Add the almond milk, cocoa powder, maple syrup, and vanilla extract to a blender and blend until smooth. Whisk in chia seeds.
- In a small bowl, gently mash the strawberries with a fork. Distribute the strawberry mash evenly to the bottom of 4 glass jars.
- Pour equal portions of the blended milk-cocoa mixture into each of the jars and let the pudding rest in the refrigerator until it achieves a pudding like consistency, at least 3 to 5 hours and up to overnight.

NUTRITION: Calories: 189; Total Fat 7g; Saturated Fat: 2g; Cholesterol: 0mg; Sodium: 60mg; Potassium: 232mg; Total Carbohydrate: 28g; Fiber: 10g; Protein: 6g

Chocolate-Mint Truffles

Preparation Time: 45 minutes
Cooking Time: 5 hours
Servings: 60 small truffles

Ingredients:
- 14 ounces semisweet chocolate, coarsely chopped
- ¾ cup half-and-half
- 1/2 teaspoon pure vanilla extract
- 1 1/2 teaspoon peppermint extract
- 2 tablespoons unsalted butter, softened
- ¾ cup naturally unsweetened or Dutch-process cocoa powder

Directions:
- Place semisweet chocolate in a large heatproof bowl.
- Microwave in four 15-second increments, stirring after each, for a total of 60 seconds. Stir until almost completely melted. Set aside.
- In a small saucepan over medium heat, heat the half-and-half, whisking occasionally, until it just begins to boil. Remove from the heat, then whisk in the vanilla and peppermint extracts.
- Pour the mixture over the chocolate and, using a wooden spoon, gently stir in one direction.

- Once the chocolate and cream are smooth, stir in the butter until it is combined and melted.
- Cover with plastic wrap pressed on the top of the mixture, and then let it sit at room temperature for 30 minutes.
- After 30 minutes, place the mixture in the refrigerator until it is thick and can hold a ball shape, about 5 hours.
- Line a large baking sheet with parchment paper or a use a silicone baking mat. Set aside.
- Remove the mixture from the refrigerator. Place the cocoa powder in a bowl.
- Scoop 1 teaspoon of the ganache and, using your hands, roll into a ball. Roll the ball in the cocoa powder, the place on the prepared baking sheet. (You can coat your palms with a little cocoa powder to prevent sticking).
- Serve immediately or cover and store at room temperature for up to 1 week.

NUTRITION: Calories: 21; Total Fat 2g; Saturated Fat: 1g; Cholesterol: 2mg; Sodium: 2mg; Potassium: 21mg; Total Carbohydrate: 2g; Fiber: 1g; Protein: 0g

Personal Mango Pies

Preparation Time: 15 minutes
Cooking Time: 14 to 16 minutes
Servings: 12

Ingredients:
- Cooking spray
- 12 small wonton wrappers
- 1 tablespoon cornstarch
- 1/2 cup water
- 3 cups finely chopped mango (fresh, or thawed from frozen, no sugar added)
- 2 tablespoons brown sugar (not packed)
- 1/2 teaspoon cinnamon
- 1 tablespoon light whipped butter or buttery spread

Directions:
- Unsweetened coconut flakes (optional)
- Preheat the oven to 350°F.
- Spray a 12-cup muffin pan with nonstick cooking spray.
- Place a wonton wrapper into each cup of the muffin pan, pressing it into the bottom and up along the sides.
- Lightly spray the wrappers with nonstick spray. Bake until lightly browned, about 8 minutes.

- Meanwhile, in a medium nonstick saucepan, combine the cornstarch with the water and stir to dissolve. Add the mango, brown sugar, and cinnamon and turn heat to medium.
- Stirring frequently, cook until the mangoes have slightly softened and the mixture is thick and gooey, 6 to 8 minutes.
- Remove the mango mixture from heat and stir in the butter.
- Spoon the mango mixture into wonton cups, about 3 tablespoons each. Top with coconut flakes (if using) and serve warm.

NUTRITION:
Calories: 61;
Total Fat 1g; S
aturated Fat: 0g;
Cholesterol: 2mg;
Sodium: 52mg;
Potassium: 77mg;
Total Carbohydrate: 14g;
Fiber: 1g;
Protein: 1g

Grilled Peach Sundaes

Preparation Time: 15 minutes
Cooking Time: 5 minutes
Servings: 1

Ingredients:

- 1 tbsp. toasted unsweetened coconut
- 1 tsp. canola oil
- 2 peaches, halved and pitted
- 2 scoops non-fat vanilla yogurt, frozen

Directions:

- Brush the peaches with oil and grill until tender.
- Place peach halves on a bowl and top with frozen yogurt and coconut.

Nutrition:
Calories: 61;
carbs: 2g;
protein: 2g;

fats: 6g;
phosphorus: 32mg;
potassium: 85mg;
sodium: 30mg

Blueberry Swirl Cake

Preparation Time: 15 minutes
Cooking Time: 45 minutes
Servings: 9

Ingredients:
- 1/2 cup margarine
- 1 1/4 cups reduced fat milk
- 1 cup granulated sugar
- 1 egg
- 1 egg white
- 1 tbsp. lemon zest, grated
- 1 tsp. cinnamon
- 1/3 cup light brown sugar
- 2 1/2 cups fresh blueberries
- 2 1/2 cups self-rising flour

Directions:
- Cream the margarine and granulated sugar using an electric mixer at high speed until fluffy.
- Add the egg and egg white and beat for another two minutes.
- Add the lemon zest and reduce the speed to low.
- Add the flour with milk alternately.
- In a greased 13x19 pan, spread half of the batter and sprinkle with blueberry on top. Add the remaining batter.
- Bake in a 350-degree Fahrenheit preheated oven for 45 minutes.
- Let it cool on a wire rack before slicing and serving.

Nutrition:
Calories: 384;
carbs: 63g;
protein: 7g;
fats: 13g;
phosphorus: 264mg;
potassium: 158mg;
sodium: 456mg

Peanut Butter Cookies

Preparation Time: 15 minutes
Cooking Time: 24 minutes
Servings: 24

Ingredients:
- 1/4 cup granulated sugar
- 1 cup unsalted peanut butter
- 1 tsp. baking soda
- 2 cups all-purpose flour
- 2 large eggs
- 2 tbsp. butter
- 2 tsp. pure vanilla extract
- 4 ounces softened cream cheese

Directions:
- Line a cookie sheet with a non-stick liner. Set aside.
- In a bowl, mix flour, sugar and baking soda. Set aside.
- On a mixing bowl, combine the butter, cream cheese and peanut butter.
- Mix on high speed until it forms a smooth consistency. Add the eggs and vanilla gradually while mixing until it forms a smooth consistency.
- Add the almond flour mixture slowly and mix until well combined.
- The dough is ready once it starts to stick together into a ball.
- Scoop the dough using a 1 tablespoon cookie scoop and drop each cookie on the prepared cookie sheet.
- Press the cookie with a fork and bake for 10 to 12 minutes at 350oF.

Nutrition:
Calories: 138;
carbs: 12g;
protein: 4g;
fats: 9g;
phosphorus: 60mg;
potassium: 84mg;
sodium: 31mg

Deliciously Good Scones

Preparation Time: 15 minutes
Cooking Time: 12 minutes
Servings: 10

Ingredients:

- 1/4 cup dried cranberries
- 1/4 cup sunflower seeds
- 1/2 teaspoon baking soda
- 1 large egg
- 2 cups all-purpose flour
- 2 tablespoon honey

Directions:

- Preheat the oven to 350oF.
- Grease a baking sheet. Set aside.
- In a bowl, mix the salt, baking soda and flour. Add the dried fruits, nuts and seeds. Set aside.
- In another bowl, mix the honey and eggs.
- Add the wet ingredients to the dry ingredients. Use your hands to mix the dough.
- Create 10 small round dough and place them on the baking sheet.
- Bake for 12 minutes.

Nutrition:
Calories: 44; carbs: 27g; protein: 4g; fats: 3g; phosphorus: 59mg; potassium: 92mg; sodium: 65mg

Mixed Berry Cobbler

Preparation Time: 15 minutes
Cooking Time: 4 hours
Servings: 8

Ingredients:

- 1/4 cup coconut milk
- 1/4 cup ghee
- 1/4 cup honey
- 1/2 cup almond flour
- 1/2 cup tapioca starch
- 1/2 tablespoon cinnamon

- 1/2 tablespoon coconut sugar
- 1 teaspoon vanilla
- 12 ounces frozen raspberries
- 16 ounces frozen wild blueberries
- 2 teaspoon baking powder
- 2 teaspoon tapioca starch

Directions:

- Place the frozen berries in the slow cooker. Add honey and 2 teaspoons of tapioca starch. Mix to combine.
- In a bowl, mix the tapioca starch, almond flour, coconut milk, ghee, baking powder and vanilla. Sweeten with sugar. Place this pastry mix on top of the berries.
- Set the slow cooker for 4 hours.

Nutrition:
Calories: 146;
carbs: 33g;
protein: 1g;
fats: 3g;
phosphorus: 29mg;
potassium: 133mg;
sodium: 4mg

Blueberry Espresso Brownies

Preparation Time: 15 minutes
Cooking Time: 30 minutes
Servings: 12

Ingredients:

- 1/4 cup organic cocoa powder
- 1/4 teaspoon salt
- 1/2 cup raw honey
- 1/2 teaspoon baking soda
- 1 cup blueberries
- 1 cup coconut cream
- 1 tablespoon cinnamon
- 1 tablespoon ground coffee

- 2 teaspoon vanilla extract
- 3 eggs

Directions:
- Preheat the oven to 3250F.
- In a bow mix together coconut cream, honey, eggs, cinnamon, honey, vanilla, baking soda, coffee and salt.
- Use a mixer to combine all ingredients.
- Fold in the blueberries
- Pour the batter in a greased baking dish and bake for 30 minutes or until a toothpick inserted in the middle comes out clean.
- Remove from the oven and let it cool.

Nutrition:
Calories: 168;
carbs: 20g;
protein: 4g;
fats: 10g;
phosphorus: 79mg;
potassium: 169mg;
sodium: 129mg

Coffee Brownies

Preparation Time: 15 minutes
Cooking Time: 20 minutes
Servings: 4

Ingredients:
- 3 eggs, beaten
- 2 tablespoons cocoa powder
- 2 teaspoons Erythritol
- 1/2 cup almond flour
- 1/2 cup organic almond milk

Directions:
- Place the eggs in the mixing bowl and combine them with Erythritol and almond milk.
- With the help of the hand mixer, whisk the liquid until homogenous.
- Then add almond flour and cocoa powder.
- Whisk the mixture until smooth.

- Take the non-sticky brownie mold and transfer the cocoa mass inside it.
- Flatten it gently with the help of the spatula. The flattened mass should be thin.
- Preheat the oven to 365F.
- Transfer the brownie in the oven and bake it for 20 minutes.
- Then chill the cooked brownies at least till the room temperature and cut into serving bars.

Nutrition:
calories 78,
fat 5.8,
fiber 1.3,
carbs 2.7,
protein 5.5

CONCLUSION

As for your well-being and health, it's a good idea to see your doctor as often as possible to make sure you don't have any preventable problems you don't need to have. The kidneys are your body's channel for toxins (as is the liver), cleaning the blood of unknown substances and toxins that are removed from things like preservatives in the food and other toxins. The moment you eat without control and fill your body with toxins, food, drink (liquor or alcohol, for example), or even the air you inhale in general, your body will also convert several things that appear to be benign until the body's organs convert them to things like formaldehyde, due to a synthetic response and transformation phase.

You likely had little knowledge about your kidneys before. You probably didn't know how you could take steps to improve your kidney health and decrease the risk of developing kidney failure. However, through reading this book, you now understand the power of the human kidney, as well as the prognosis of chronic kidney disease. While over thirty-million Americans are being affected by kidney disease, you can now take steps to be one of the people who is actively working to promote your kidney health.

These stats are alarming, which is why it is necessary to take proper care of your kidneys, starting with a kidney-friendly diet. These recipes are ideal whether you have been diagnosed with a kidney problem or you want to prevent any kidney issue. This isn't a condition that occurs without any forethought; it is a dynamic issue and in that it very well may be both found early and treated, diet changed, and settling what is causing the issue is conceivable. It's conceivable to have partial renal failure yet, as a rule; it requires some time (or downright poor diet for a short time) to arrive at absolute renal failure. You would prefer not to reach total renal failure since this will require standard dialysis treatments to save your life.

One such case is a large part of the dietary sugars used in diet sodas - for example, aspartame is converted to formaldehyde in the body. These toxins must be excreted or they can cause disease, renal (kidney) failure, malignant growth, and various other painful problems

Dialysis treatments explicitly clean the blood of waste and toxins in the blood utilizing a machine in light of the fact that your body can no longer carry out the responsibility. Without treatments, you could die a very painful death. Renal failure can be the consequence of long-haul diabetes, hypertension, unreliable diet, and can stem from other health concerns. A renal diet is tied in with directing the intake of protein and phosphorus in your eating routine. Restricting your sodium intake is likewise significant. By controlling these two variables you can control the vast majority of the toxins/waste made by your body, enabling your kidney to 100% function. In the event that you get this early enough and truly moderate your diets with extraordinary consideration, you could avert complete renal failure. If you get this early, you can take out the issue completely.

Manufactured by Amazon.ca
Bolton, ON